Fight Fat, Fight Fatigue
Energy Makeover

THE **Sun***Slimmer*

Fight Fat, Fight Fatigue
Energy Makeover

Sally Ann Voak and Nicki Waterman

Thorsons

Thorsons
An Imprint of HarperCollins*Publishers*
77–85 Fulham Palace Road,
Hammersmith, London W6 8JB

The Thorsons website address is: www.thorsons.com

and *Thorsons*
are trademarks of
HarperCollins*Publishers*

Published by Thorsons 2002

10 9 8 7 6 5 4 3 2

© Nicki Waterman and Sally Ann Voak 2002

Nicki Waterman and Sally Ann Voak assert the moral right to be
identified as the authors of this work

A catalogue record for this book
is available from the British Library

ISBN 0 00 711868 6

Photography by Steve Lewis

Printed and bound in Great Britain by
Martins the Printers Ltd, Berwick upon Tweed

CONTENTS

INTRODUCTION

Feeling stressed out, tired and utterly fed up with trying to find the answer to your yo-yo weight problems?

Stop trying to deal with these as separate issues, and tackle fatigue and fat together. That's the easiest and most effective way to get into great shape.

There have been many books written about how to lose weight, and quite a few about beating tiredness – but *Fight Fat, Fight Fatigue* is the very first practical workbook that tells you how to do both.

In fact, the two problems go hand in hand.

Think about it: if you are overweight, you are forcing your body (your limbs and your organs such as your heart, liver, kidneys) to work harder. You are certainly eating badly as well. So, you are bound to feel more tired. Even if you are only carrying 10 kilos (a stone and a half) of excess weight, you are putting your body under unnecessary strain.

Similarly, if you are suffering from excessive tiredness, your body has to work harder just to perform everyday functions like walking, working, talking and even sleeping. It is well known that feeling fatigued makes you crave more sugary, fatty foods in order to raise your flagging blood sugar level. As a result, you are very likely to put on excess weight.

Before you know what's hit you, you are caught in a vicious circle: you eat more to stay on top of your daily life, yet carry more weight which, in turn, makes you less active and less lively.

The good news is that once you can unlock the secret of how to eat properly and exercise correctly, both problems will, like the fat on your body, just melt away!

The two authors of this book, *Sun* Slimming Editor Sally Ann Voak and fitness trainer Nicki Waterman, have come up with a winning formula for fighting fat and fatigue.

Between them Sally and Nicki have had many years' experience of helping overweight, stressed, tired people to shape up ... and they can do the same for you. They have very different backgrounds, but one important thing in common: they both believe that there is no need to spend a fortune or become a fitness fanatic to feel great. Their practical approach made them a winning team with the thousands of *Sun* readers and GMTV viewers who ask their advice every day.

During the newspaper's regular 'hotlines', where readers phone in for confidential advice, the twin demons of fat and fatigue are a common problem, particularly for women who have children and a job, and men who are trying to make it in the tough workplace and still spend 'quality' time with their family and friends. Sally and Nicki help callers to take the first steps towards improving things, whether they need to make simple lifestyle changes or get expert help with serious medical or mental health problems.

The two women are very different, in age and lifestyle: Sally has been married for 38 years and is the mother of two grown-up sons. Acknowledged as Britain's leading nutrition journalist, she has been writing on diet and health subjects for *The Sun* for 30 years. This is her 28th book. She is 5 ft 6 in tall, weighs 8 st 10 lb, and is more active now than she has ever been in her life.

Nicki is 39, with a 17-year-old daughter and 15-year-old son. She lives with her partner of six years. Until 12 years ago she faced a constant struggle to stay in shape, and had a nagging weight problem. Then (as you will read in Chapter 1), she discovered the benefits of exercise. Now she is one of the country's top fitness trainers. Among her showbiz clients are the former members of the pop sensation All Saints, and she is a regular on GMTV's morning programme. She is 5 ft 3 in tall and now weighs a steady 7 st 7 lb.

Sally and Nicki are delighted to share their wealth of knowledge with YOU.

You may be asking, will their ideas work for me?

Well, as always, our two experts believe in putting their theories to the test. So, they enlisted six overweight, stressed out, tired 'guinea pigs', aged 20 to 57, with very different lifestyles, to try the Fight Fat, Fight Fatigue programme over a period of three months.

In total, our volunteers lost 87 lb. They all feel wonderful, and are having a lot of fun enjoying their new, slimmer shape and high energy levels.

The Fight Fat, Fight Fatigue programme worked brilliantly for them. It will work just as brilliantly for you. And that's a promise.

CHAPTER ONE

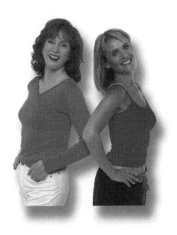

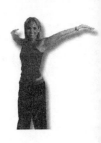

WHY YOU NEED US!

C an you pinch more than an inch around your waistline? Do you have to pinch YOURSELF to stay awake during a boring afternoon at your work-station or while you are doing the household chores?

If you do, you are not alone. These are problems that are familiar to all of us. Sadly, we've become a nation of overweight, stressed, tired people who have to struggle through the day just to get everything done.

Most people's response to fatigue is to eat high-fat foods and drink alcohol. At the end of an exhausting week, it's so tempting to crash out in front of the TV with a takeaway, or drown your sorrows over a few bevvies in the pub with your mates. As will be demonstrated in this book, obesity exacerbates tiredness, so the problem of tiredness gets worse ... not better.

WHAT CAN BE DONE?

It's easy for pundits to say 'Change your lifestyle' or 'Pull your socks up.'

The latest TV advertisements even use shock tactics to jolt us into health awareness, such as a graphic image of an overweight father succumbing to a heart attack in a busy shopping precinct. The clear message is 'Watch out – if you don't shape up, you'll die young.'

These tactics do hit hard, but do they work? Unfortunately, the vast majority of people prefer to pretend that the health pundits are talking about someone else – and reach for another biscuit or can of beer.

Our approach is very different. We believe that getting into shape and eating properly should be FUN. Our own experience has proved that you can still enjoy the good things in life like a drink in the pub, or the occasional pizza in front of the TV if your general lifestyle is a healthy one. That doesn't mean being a fitness fanatic and living on brown rice and lettuce leaves – perish the thought! It simply means making subtle changes which will reap incredible rewards.

A GROWING PROBLEM

People often ask us why the population is getting fatter and lazier when there are more gyms and fitness clubs in this country than ever before, when the range of healthy foods available has never been greater, and when our role models are superslim film stars and superfit athletes.

There are two answers to this question. The obvious one is that we are surrounded by temptation, and have so many worries that we haven't got the time or energy to take ourselves in hand. The second answer is even more obvious, but much more difficult to face up to. The sad fact is that, in the Western world (and increasingly in the East) 21st-century humans are becoming more like robots than people who can make up their own minds. Our original function as hunters and warriors ceased to exist centuries ago, so we no longer have to live on our wits just to get through another dangerous day. Everything is done for us, so instead of taking control of our own lives, we live vicariously through media images on TV, the internet and in glossy magazines. It's so much easier to watch a TV programme or read an article about healthy eating, than it is to shop for and prepare a nutritious meal. It's far simpler to enrol at a gym and let the membership lapse than to make the effort actually to use the facilities a couple of times a week, and it's much more pleasant to read about a famous person's slimming or fitness success than to get off your backside and work out. Sad, isn't it?

But, it doesn't have to be like that. You can choose to be different! In Chapter 2 you will be introduced to six people who, when we met them, weren't exactly robots (yet!), but were beginning to think that they were destined to spend the rest of their lives being overweight and tired all the time. They wanted to change, but didn't know how.

Like our volunteers, you also want to change, and you have made the first move towards enjoying a new, fitter lifestyle by buying this book. Will you read it once and then put it on a shelf, or will you take our advice? Hopefully, you will be inspired to follow the programme properly for at least three months, and to use it as the basis for a lifetime of healthy living. We hope you do, and that you will contact us (at the address on page 153) to let us know how you get on.

BEFORE YOU START

Before embarking on any major lifestyle change, it is a good idea to have a medical check-up. It is absolutely essential to do so if you are very overweight (BMI of more than 40 – more about this on page 10 – or a waist measurement of more than 34½ inches [women] or 40 inches [men]), have diabetes, suffer from heart disease, respiratory problems, or have any other illness or condition which could make it hazardous to alter your daily eating and exercise routine.

Most medical practices now have 'Well Woman' and 'Well Man' clinics where you can get the advice you need, and you could also arrange to have regular check-ups to monitor important health indicators such as weight, blood-pressure, cholesterol levels, lung function, etc. This is important because weight loss alone is NOT an indication that you are improving your fitness level (in fact, it could indicate the opposite). Our six volunteers all underwent rigorous health screening before and after taking part in our Fight Fat, Fight Fatigue (FFFF) programme.

BE REALISTIC ABOUT YOUR AIMS

The goal of this programme is to provide a healthy diet and exercise programme which you can maintain on a day-to-day basis without sacrificing your life for it. You want to shed weight, but this isn't just about jumping on the scales every few days. Instead, take a good look at yourself in the mirror and check out your basic shape. After years of working with overweight, unfit people, we are both very realistic about our bodies: Sally is tallish, with a narrow frame, slim hips and a small bust. Excess weight tends to accumulate around her stomach (she is a classic 'apple' shape). Nicki is exactly the opposite: petite, but shaped rather like a dumb-bell – wide on both ends and slim in the middle. If she gains weight, it goes straight on her upper legs.

If you are a large woman with a big frame, you are never going to look fragile. If you are a very petite woman, you are never going to look like an Olympic swimmer, with big shoulders and long legs. If you are a short, fat man, you are not, miraculously, going to turn into a Greek God. Our aim is not to give you a body to die for, but a body to live for ... in other words, the very best of *you*.

MOTIVATION

While you are following the Fight Fat, Fight Fatigue programme (and afterwards!), it's vital to keep yourself highly motivated. If you have a partner who is encouraging, that can be helpful. But YOU must be the prime mover. You can do this in several ways:

1 **Practise some positive visualization techniques.**

Sit quietly in your bedroom or sitting room. Now relax, breathe evenly and close your eyes. Imagine yourself looking fit and attractive in a setting that evokes peace and fun: a tropical beach, a country park, on a mountain. You feel full of energy, ready for anything, and very happy indeed. Let yourself enjoy the scene, and your own part in it, for a few minutes before you open your eyes and return to the real world. Keep this image, and your own special 'place' in your mind, and return there from time to time during your diet and fitness programme.

2 **Keep a diary of your progress.**

It can be a simple weekly update if you like, noting your weight, how you feel, and what benefits you have noticed from your new lifestyle.

3 **Think ahead – to your next holiday, wedding, party or other special event.**

Plan just what you will be wearing, and how good you will look (use those visualization techniques again). Whenever you feel tempted to skip your daily walk, or forget about eating breakfast, think about the event ahead and how you will look and feel. No, this isn't selfish – it is practical and positive.

TAKING CONTROL

Let's introduce you to the 'Big Four' 21st-century Fat and Fatigue hazards, and how to deal with them.

These are the four things that people blame most often for their wobbly bodies and lack of energy. What they fail to recognize is that what counts is not the actual hazard itself, but our response to it, and the way we deal with the problem.

We want you to focus on being in control. So, before embarking on our programme, read our practical tips for 'conditioning' yourself to respond positively to even the most negative influences. Our ideas will help you to start your new diet and exercise routines with confidence. *You **can** do it!*

1. Fast Food

FACTS

Yes, fast food is here to stay. Yes, there is a burger bar on every high street, and supermarket ready-meals are turning us all into lazybones.

But just hang on a minute. Although we are in the grip of junk-food fever, all is not doom and gloom. It is also true that there has never been such a wide variety of healthy, fresh food available. Whether you choose organic or not, the supermarkets offer a huge range of seasonal, fresh foods; farmers' markets where local-grown produce is sold are springing up all over the country, and you can now buy almost anything you want at a reasonable price.

ACTION

Ignore the hype, and decide what you and your family want to eat and where you want to eat it. Use our menus (see Chapter 4) to help you plan a good basic diet that's easy to prepare. Enjoy shopping, and always take a list so you don't get side-tracked by the latest 'special offer'. Take a packed lunch to work if the canteen is rubbish, and always keep fruit in your car when you travel long distances. If you want an occasional junk-food meal, eat it without guilt.

2. Sedentary Living

We are becoming a nation of couch potatoes, and even schoolchildren are at risk of developing heart disease because of their sedentary lifestyles. The only kind of exercise many people bother with is surfing the internet. The car rules the world, and nothing anyone can do (particularly the politicians) will persuade people to give up their womb-like motors and use public transport or even – horrors – walk! Some pessimists even believe that humans will gradually lose the use of their legs, and become short, fat, stumpy beings who are permanently connected to their mobile phones or computers.

ACTION

In our experience, vague promises to 'walk more' or 'leave the car at home sometimes' don't work. Instead, set yourself a daily target to walk briskly for 20 minutes. You can do it first thing in the morning, like Nicki, during the day (at lunchtime, perhaps) or when you come home in the evening. Wear comfortable shoes, swing your arms and march purposefully, working up to a pace of about 6.2–6.5 kilometres per hour, so that in your 20 minutes you cover a distance of about 2–2.16 km. (That's fast enough to feel a bit puffed, but not so fast that you can't hold a conversation if you persuade a partner to come along!) By all means, join a gym if you can afford to, but make sure you get your money's worth by going regularly. Numerous studies have shown that people who get up early and work out at the gym in the morning stick to their routine more easily than those who go at night. So, it's important to find a gym near your home or work. Finally, find a sporting activity that you enjoy, such as swimming or cycling, which you can fit into your weekly schedule.

3. Stress

Life is getting more difficult. At any rate, that is how we perceive it. It's certainly true that stress levels are rocketing. Emails are popping up all day long, there's pressure to work long hours, pressure to rush everywhere, pressure, pressure, pressure. Far from helping us get more leisure time, modern technology seems to drive us to work harder, and produces more problems. Isn't it amazing, too, the way modern machines 'gang up' on us? If one goes wrong, they all do! There are other stress-inducing pressures too: we are expected to look good, run a wonderful home (immaculately decorated), raise perfect children, and enjoy fantastic sex with a caring partner. If only!

ACTION

We need to get things in proportion. If you feel stressed out, take a good look at your life and work out which aspects are producing this stress. Are you an alcoholic, or near alcoholic (see below)? Are your relationship problems too difficult to solve alone? Are you so depressed that you feel as though you have a big, black cloud over your head? You can get marvellous professional help for any of these problems, and there is a list of useful contact numbers and addresses on page 149. Use them.

If your job is stressful, look at the reasons why – write them down. Is the journey to and from your workplace eating into your day? Are your colleagues upsetting you? Is the workload impossible to complete within sensible hours? You only have one life, so tackle these things sensibly by talking about them. If it's practical, even think about changing your job.

Maybe, like so many people, you simply feel that the various elements of your life – work, home responsibilities, socializing – add up to a demanding daily schedule that is just impossible to cope with. Prioritize, get more help (from friends, family), be less conscientious. Make some time every day for yourself: listen to music, read, talk to a friend. As you will find out in Chapter 6, exercise is one of the best ways to beat stress. Of course, a healthy diet is vitally important, too.

Fight Fat, Fight Fatigue

4. Alcohol

FACTS

We are a nation of boozers, and drink-related illnesses such as cirrhosis, hepatitis, strokes and cancer are increasing every year. In the past it has been men who did most of the drinking, but now women are catching up fast and it affects them more. Women tend to weigh less and have a higher proportion of fat on their bodies, so anything they drink is more concentrated.

Let's be honest about it – alcohol is a drug, and a poison. It is very fattening, stops us absorbing essential vitamins, and makes us tired and stupid. It is dangerous because it is socially acceptable to be a drinker. There are enormous opportunities to drink –theme pubs, clubs and winebars are incredibly profitable, so they are springing up everywhere, especially near railway stations and shopping centres, and home booze consumption is going through the roof. Enough said.

ACTION

Make a list of all the drinks you have in a week and where you have them, and who with. It is a myth that alcoholics drink alone. As you know by now, the 'safe' limit for men is 27 units, for women 21 units per week (one unit is the equivalent of half a pint of beer, or a 'short' drink or a glass of wine). If your total is above that, have a big think. Do you need help? Addiction (to booze, food, sex, gambling, etc.), is a common problem, and nothing to be ashamed of. There's a list of numbers to ring on page 151.

If you are confident that your drinking is out of habit or social circumstances, do something about it. Have at least three or four booze-free days a week, limit weekend boozing, and drink water with meals when you are served wine. Enjoy the feeling of clearheadedness, the longer days, the alertness. Plus, of course, the twin bonuses: weight loss, and energy gain.

Why you need us!

Nicki and Sally are both women who enjoy the occasional drink. Recently, Nicki decided that her workload of writing, TV and personal appearances was so heavy that she needed to be in top form all the time, so she has stopped drinking any alcohol for the time being. However, she will be sipping the occasional glass of red wine again, soon! Sally limits drinking to the 'safe' unit level or below, and aims for three or four days weekly without alcohol. Her favourite tipple is stout (100 calories per half pint), which she enjoys as a mineral-rich nutritional booster, as well as a refreshing drink.

HOW ARE FAT AND FATIGUE AFFECTING YOUR LIFE?

Try this quiz to find out more about your own overweight and tiredness levels, and how they are affecting your ability to change your lifestyle and get in shape.
Tick A, B or C for each question, and see your results, below.

1 What is your Body Mass Index measurement?
You calculate this by dividing your weight in kilograms by your height in metres, squared. For example, if you weigh 66 kilos (10 st 5 lb) and are 1.72 metres (5 ft 7 in) tall, you can work out your BMI by dividing 66 by 2.8 (which is 1.72, squared). Your BMI works out at 23.5.

Once you have calculated your BMI, check it against this list:

- Below 20: Underweight
- 20–25: Acceptable Weight Range
- 25–30: Overweight
- 30–40: Obese
- Over 40: Very Obese

A: Are you within the acceptable or just within the overweight range?
B: Towards the upper end of the overweight range, or lower end of obese?
C: Obese or very obese?

2   What is your waist measurement?

Women:
A: Less than 80 cm (31½ in)
B: Between 80 and 88 cm (31½ and 34 in)
C: Over 88 cm (34½ in)

Men:
A: Less than 94 cm (37 in)
B: Between 94 and 102 cm (37 and 40 in)
C: Over 102 cm (40 in)

3   How many hours' sleep do you have each night?
A: Between 6 and 8 hours
B: Between 8 and 10 hours
C: Between 2 and 6 hours

4   How much exercise do you take?
A: At least 20 minutes of brisk exercise three times a week, plus regular gym work-outs, swimming, sports
B: Daily walking, housework, swimming on holiday
C: As little as possible

5   At which time of day is fatigue most likely to be a problem?
A: Late evening
B: After lunch or mid-afternoon
C: Mid-morning or lunchtime

6   Which of these is most like your own daily eating pattern?
A: Three healthy meals a day, plus fruit and sometimes chocolate or biscuits for snacks, and the occasional alcoholic drink
B: No breakfast, sandwich lunch, snacks of crisps and fruit in the afternoon, proper family dinner at night

Why you need us!

C: No set mealtimes, instead you snack on fast food, takeaways and high-fat nibbles at irregular times throughout the day

7   How many units of alcohol do you drink each week? (A unit is half a pint of beer or lager, or a pub-measure short drink, or a glass of wine)
    A: less than 25
    B: 25–35
    C: more than 35

8   Which of the following foods do you crave when you feel tired?
    A: Fruit – especially bananas
    B: Cereals, bread
    C: Biscuits, crisps, cakes

9   How do you react if you have to perform an unexpected energetic task – running for a bus, for instance?
    A: Annoyed, but ready to make a dash
    B: Panicky
    C: I don't run for buses

10 Has your partner or a close member of your family ever commented about your size?
    A: Only in a complimentary way
    B: In a joking fashion, when out shopping or looking through holiday snaps
    C: They wouldn't dare!

11 How would you describe your libido?
    A: Healthy, thank you
    B: I feel sexier on holiday and at weekends
    C: Food is the new sex

12 Which of these descriptions best fits your parents?
> **A:** They were slim and sporty when young, but thickened out in
> middle age
>
> **B:** They were quite chunky, and took little exercise
>
> **C:** They were very fat, and that's why I'm fat, too

13 Which of these descriptions is closest to your own image of yourself?
> **A:** Fairly attractive, but I could look better and feel fitter
>
> **B:** However hard I try to be positive, the mirror tells me I'm
> chubby and tired-looking
>
> **C:** I never look in mirrors

Mostly A

You are well on the way to achieving the perfect weight and fitness level for your body type and lifestyle. Three months on our diet and exercise plan will make a tremendous difference to your vitality, and help you lose that excess flab. Many people who are just like you – not exactly unhealthy, but not bouncing with brilliance, either –would be happy to settle back and let age, and weight, creep on. You are different. Well done. Enjoy the positive changes that are in store for you.

Mostly B

Buying this book was your first step towards a slimmer, healthier future. You are, quite rightly, worried about your size, and the health problems associated with being overweight. Although you have probably tried to slim down and shape up before, you are not a failure. Forget all those 'hiccups', and start again. It is never too late to make positive changes and, once you start to enjoy your new lifestyle, the rewards are tremendous. The first thing to remember is that, with our help, YOU CAN DO IT.

Why you need us!

Mostly C

You must realize that you have serious problems, but the big challenge is to do something about them. You should have a medical check-up before starting our programme and, if possible, get your doctor to monitor your progress with regular weigh-ins. The most important thing of all is your mental attitude: you must be willing to change the bad habits of a lifetime. Are you? If you have doubts about this, then counselling sessions can help. There is a list of specialist counselling organizations on page 151.

BREAKOUT

Double Act – Sally and Nicki Confess!

OK, guys and girls, let's get the record straight. We would be the first to admit that we haven't stayed in shape by resting on our laurels. But, we'll let you into a little secret. We are both happier with our bodies and our lives than we have ever been. Our body fat is evenly distributed to give us a soft, feminine look. Our hair is shiny, our skin has a glow, our energy levels are incredible and we can focus on many different things ... being with partners and children, love for the theatre and art, for instance ... or the simple pleasures of a sunset or visit to a gallery.

SALLY

'My personal experience is that life really does get better as you get older. Of course I have been lucky to be involved in writing about health and nutrition for so long ... by this time, I must have learned something! The positive power of a healthy diet (which includes some alcohol, and yes, even the odd pizza or two) has always been fascinating to me, and I am very conscious of eating regular balanced meals. However, I must confess that, when I was younger I was never very keen on exercise, apart from swimming. It's only in the last two years that I have discovered that stepping up the action to include regular work-outs at the gym really does help me stay in shape more easily and is great fun as well. Now, my twice-weekly fitness routine and long weekend walks are nearly as important to my overall wellbeing as my low-fat diet.

'It's just as well that I feel so energetic, because my schedule is more hectic than ever. My two sons are grown up and married, but my husband and I are still incredibly busy. I'm enjoying my work, home, travelling, the theatre, opera, skiing, swimming, rugby (as a club Vice President, not a player!), socializing with friends and family. There simply aren't enough hours in the day to pack in all the pleasures that life has to offer.

'As far as my figure is concerned, well that's fine too. OK, so I will never have a completely flat stomach, my legs are too thin, and my boobs too small, but I'm a neat size 10, I have more vitality than most 25-year-olds and, overall, I feel good about myself. If this is middle age, great!'

15

NICKI

'If someone had tried to tell me 12 years ago when I was struggling with my weight that fitness would be this easy today, I would have laughed. To tell the truth, I was scared to death to even start. I was afraid that I would have to spend five hours a day working out and eat like a bird if I wanted to end up looking like some gorgeous supermodel on the front cover of a magazine. Then I read somewhere that muscle had "memory" and that even when you're not training hard your body will remember how to maintain its shape. That sounded like pie in the sky to me, but 12 years later I'm writing this book with Sally to tell you that it's true ... and to show you how easy it is to get in shape and feel energized. Now, as far as pumping iron is concerned, the only heavyweight in my life is Hugo, my pet bearded collie dog. Speedwalking and light weight-training keep me in shape, and my mirror and my favourite jeans are all I need to "measure" my progress. If my cheeks don't look like a chipmunk's, and my jeans zip up without a struggle, I know I am within my "optimum" weight range.

'I am on the move all day long, keeping up with my two fabulous children and my partner, my social life and my work. Some weeks I'm even too busy to exercise! Like Sally, I have so much fun that I want to share my recipe for happiness with others. If I can do it, you can do it too.'

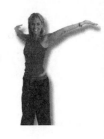

CHAPTER TWO

MEET OUR FIGHTERS

There is only one way to prove that any diet and exercise regime really works, and that is to try it out. We did just that. We found six volunteers who were all, in various ways, fighting the twin problems of overweight and excessive tiredness.

They are different ages and lead different lives, but when you read through their stories you are sure to recognize many of your own symptoms. Before recruiting our 'guinea pigs', we chatted to them about their daily routines and we found that, despite their differences, they all had one important thing in common: a strong feeling that they weren't getting the most out of life. Let's face it, you can have all the money and love in the world, but if you feel unfit and are not happy with your body, you are missing out. Our gang were bowling along, coping adequately (as we all try to do), but knew, deep down, that they would be able to cope better and enjoy themselves much more if they were fitter.

Before they started our programme, we put our six through a fitness test, to check out their heart rate, lung function and general levels of fitness. This is a good idea for anyone who is making serious changes to their lifestyle.

(There is a contact number for organizing a private test on page 156.)

Each volunteer – five women and one man – was given a 'prescription' and we monitored their progress closely for three months with regular weigh-ins, counselling sessions, and group 'fun runs' and exercise sessions. As one of them, hairdresser Lydia, said it was 'a bit like joining the army, but with a couple of nagging lady field marshalls in charge, instead of good-looking blokes'. Sorry, Lydia, but we never bullied ... we just coaxed you into action!

The five women in our team were all in what Nicki politely called a 'deconditioned state', so their training heart rates were set at a slightly lower pace than our lone male volunteer, who works as a builder and was already in fairly good shape.

An important part of our volunteers' programme was cardiovascular exercise. At a gym you would probably be shown how to monitor your own heart rate, but Nicki provided a very easy way of determining how hard you are working your heart:

While you are exercising (running, walking, cycling, swimming), imagine your exertions on a scale of 1 to 10.

Level 1 is easy (i.e. you can chat happily to a pal while you exercise, and keep going for a long time).
Between **Levels 2 and 4**, you are making more effort.
Level 5 is still moderately easy (you can still chat, but it is more difficult, and you can't keep going for ever!).
Between **Levels 6 and 8**, you are working much harder.
Once you get to **Level 9**, it is impossible to hold a conversation.
Level 10 is hard (you are out of breath and feel shattered afterwards).

Here are details of our gang, their eating patterns and fitness levels before starting Sally's diet and Nicki's exercise routine, and the prescription we gave for each of them.

LYDIA

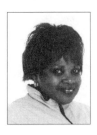

Age: 30
Height: 5ft 2½in
Starting Weight: 11 st 6
  (160lbs/73 kg)
Job: Hairdresser

Waist: 38 in
Tummy: 36in
Buttocks: 40in
Body Fat %: 39.3% (very high)
Blood Pressure: 135/86
Lung Function: 75% (normal)

Single girl Lydia lives in a flat in North London and works as a hair-dresser at Strawberry Hair Studio, a top salon. Her clients include our Nicki, and former *Coronation Street* star Beverley Callard.

There's no doubt that hairdressing is one of the most tiring profes-sions of all. It is difficult to eat properly because local salons are often in high streets where there are fast-food joints. It is all too tempting to grab a burger or send out for a slab of pizza if you are very busy. Lydia spends long hours on her feet every day, except on Sunday and Monday, which are her days off. Just before she started her FFFF course, Lydia had been ill with backache suffered after long hours of blow-drying clients' hair during the pre-Christmas rush. She was so tired and run down that she was spending practically all of her time off in bed, or fast asleep on the sofa!

Lydia's weight had gradually crept up over the past five years through 'comfort eating':

"I admit that I am the first person to turn to junk food if I am tired or upset. I've had a number of family tragedies over the last few years. Mum passed away six years ago, and I still haven't come to terms with my grief. Three years ago my uncle, who was very close to mum and helped bring me up, died as well. When I'm feeling tired after a hard Saturday in the hair salon, and a bit tearful, the easiest way to cheer myself up is with a big meal and a few drinks.

I played lacrosse, netball and rounders at school, but gave them up when I went to hairdressing college. Now, I just don't have time for sport. I spend an hour and a half travelling to and from work every day, and am shattered on my day off.

I mean to look after myself better, but my good intentions go out of the window."

Like all our volunteers, Lydia was asked to fill in a 'Food Diary' before starting our programme. This revealed that she rarely ate breakfast, snacked on a tuna and salad roll or some soup at lunchtime, and then ate a Chinese takeaway or chicken and chips for supper. Most evenings she was drinking a couple of brandies or a few glasses of wine, and on Saturday night she often had a boozy binge at a party. Exercise was sporadic: the occasional long walk, a half-hearted session at the gym. Not surprisingly, under the 'Comment' section in her diary her most frequent remark was 'very tired'.

Our Prescription for Lydia

DIET

Sally: Although her daily calorie intake was too high (about 3,000 daily), Lydia's diet was seriously low in iron, which is one of the most common causes of fatigue. It's been estimated that about a quarter of all women of childbearing age are iron-deficient, so this is not an unusual problem. The best sources of iron are meat, fortified breakfast cereals, beans, nuts, seeds and eggs. To aid iron absorption it's necessary to take in sufficient vitamin C, in fresh fruit and vegetables, and Lydia's diet was low in both. She rarely ate breakfast, had a very light lunch, and most of her calories were taken in late at night, when her work was over. Her evening meal choices were fat-loaded as well.

Her diet was also low in the vitamin B group, which is something that often occurs with people who consume quite a lot of alcohol and don't eat many dairy products, eggs, or vegetables. Vitamin B_1 (thiamin) and Vitamin B_{12} are particularly associated with tiredness.

Lydia needed a much more structured and sensible approach to eating. I put her on our diet programme (see Chapter 8), and made her keep food diaries for three months to ensure that she stuck to the plan. She also cut her alcohol intake down by about a half (about 20 units weekly), drank more water and mineral water, and ate regularly instead of skipping meals.

EXERCISE

Nicki: It was vital for Lydia to strengthen her lower back (*erector spinae*), as she stands all day long while hairdressing. Sit-ups helped to balance her physique, and T'ai Chi has had a beneficial effect on her posture, leaving her feeling much better at the end of her working day. For the first six weeks I recommended 30 minutes of cardiovascular exercise daily (running, cycling) each day at level 5–6, plus brisk walking alternating with power walking, swimming (four slow lengths, one fast length) and lower back and T'ai Chi exercises.

During the second six weeks, Lydia increased the cardiovascular work to 45 minutes a day, at level 7–9 on four days a week, and walking was intensified up to jogging level. She continued with her lower back exercises, and added sit-ups and crunches (three sets of 15–20 repetitions) to complement her back exercises. T'ai Chi for relaxation completed the second half of her programme.

21

ALAN

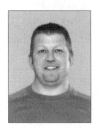

Age: 43	Waist: 35 in
Height: 5ft 10in	Tummy: 38 in
Starting Weight: 14 st 7	Buttocks: 39 in
(203 lb/92 kg)	Body Fat %: normal
Job: Builder and Student	Blood Pressure: 150/90
Chest: 44 in	Lung Function: 80% (good)

Alan, from Stevenage, Herts, is a good-looking guy who works very hard as a builder and is also studying for an MA degree in Literary Studies. He is divorced, with a 20-year-old son and two daughters aged 17 and 13.

When we met Alan he was feeling tired and stressed out, and had nearly given up on achieving the 'six-pack' chest he longed for.

"I've put on weight as I've got older, and assumed that my metabolism has slowed down. Up until the age of 25, I played hockey, football and rugby regularly, but when my building business took off I had to work all the hours I could, and there just wasn't time to take part in team games.

My daily routine is fairly simple. I get up at 6 a.m., eat some cereal for breakfast, then I make some sandwiches to take to work, together with fruit and crisps. I drive to my work site, which is usually within a 40 mile radius of my home, then spend the day climbing ladders and heaving bricks around. It is tiring work and I allow myself a half-hour break for my sandwiches at midday and continue until about 5 p.m. I cook myself a dinner when I get home, which could be anything from chops to fish and chips. I might have a few pints on a Saturday night, but generally do not drink very much beer.

It is very hard to motivate yourself to spend an hour working out after a long day and when you know that you have assignments to write for college as well. I must fit in at least 10 hours on my course-work each week to get my degree. This is very important to me, as I have always been keen on literature, and didn't have a chance to take a degree when I was younger. I've even had poetry published, and written three chapters of a novel. You've only got one life, and I intend to enjoy mine to the full."

As well as improving his physique, Alan wanted to know where he could find extra energy to keep him alert for study.

Our Prescription for Alan

DIET

Sally: Like so many men approaching middle age, Alan thought he could eat the same foods as when he was younger, without spreading. The sad fact is that most men become less active (and Alan, although a builder by trade, certainly was less active than he had been at 25) as they age, but carry on eating the same foods, and drink more alcohol. Sorry, fellas, there really is no such thing as 'middle-age spread' ... it's just the result of over-indulgence and lack of activity.

Luckily, Alan is not a big boozer, so it was quite easy to tailor our diet plan to fit in with his new, fitter lifestyle. He needed more carbohydrate to fuel his muscles for work and exercise. His breakfast was inadequate, so I advised him to add more toast, extra fruit and the occasional low-fat cooked meal to his early morning menus. To make his lunch more interesting, he stocked up with pitta bread, vegetable soups, and experimented with some of my suggestions for sandwich fillings. He also allowed time for a mid-afternoon snack as well, to give him the energy to work out or study in the early evening. Cooking for one isn't always easy, but he quickly started experimenting with my easy supper recipes, and switched from chips to jacket potatoes.

Meet our fighters

EXERCISE

Nicki: Alan was already very fit, but he needed to increase cardiovascular work in order to get rid of his 'love handles'. Weight-training sessions helped to maintain his muscle mass and keep him toned, and T'ai Chi exercises prevented him from becoming 'muscle bound' by improving his flexibility. For the first six weeks he spent 40–45 minutes a day on cardiovascular work, aiming for level 6–8. I recommended moderately energetic jogging with 30-second sprints of intensity. He went to an aero-skip class (combining aerobics and skipping rope work to intensify the workout) and took in some weight-training in his local gym plus my T'ai Chi exercises.

During the second six weeks of our three-month programme, he increased his cardiovascular workout to level 7–9, pushing up his jogging level to higher intensity, and carried on with the aero-skip, weight-training and T'ai Chi.

JAIE

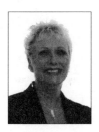

Age: 41
Height: 5ft 3 in
Starting Weight: 12 st
 (168 lb/76 kg
Job: Beauty Consultant
Bust: 38½ in

Waist: 31 in
Tummy: 32 in
Buttocks: 42 in
Body Fat %: 30.75%
Blood Pressure: 124/90
Lung Function: 75% (normal)

Jaie is a very attractive, hard-working mum who is married to Dave, 38, a businessman. The couple have two daughters – Lauren, 14, and Chloe, 4 – and live in Welling, Kent. On the surface, Jaie appears to be a very dynamic, energetic woman. Her job, as a cosmetics consultant, demands a high standard of grooming, and Jaie certainly looks the part. Timid clients who might be overawed by her immaculate appearance will be cheered to know that Jaie isn't total perfection; indeed, like so many women, she has been a 'yo-yo' dieter all her life.

25

"It all started when I was a teenager. I was never satisfied with my shape, and spent my life going on the latest 'fad' diets … and failing to stick to them. Nine years ago, I lost about 10 lb in four weeks, and trimmed down to 9 st. I felt great, but the weight gradually crept back on.

I can always raise plenty of energy for work. But at the end of the day, I tend to collapse like a deflated balloon. I just wish my fat tummy did the same thing … it seems to expand as the day goes on.

I often hold social gatherings for my work-mates, and they tease me by calling me the 'cheesecake' queen because I eat so much of it. I absolutely love butter, as well, and eat so much of it that my thighs look like blobs of the stuff. With all my dieting knowledge, I know that you've got to cut fat to shed weight, but somehow I can't do it. I love a few drinks with my friends, too, and at weekends I might consume a couple of bottles of wine."

Meet our fighters

Our Prescription for Jaie

DIET

Sally: Jaie is suffering from the same problem that affects all 'yo-yo' dieters: her body has become used to a 'feast or famine' situation, and now when she does try to slim down it is very difficult to do so. Quite sensibly, when there's a 'famine' her brain tells her body to react by storing energy carefully. I advised Jaie to stop worrying about her weight, and concentrate on eating properly. Her high intake of fat is dangerous: heart disease is now the most common cause of death in women. She also experiences uncomfortable fluid retention, so I advised her to cut back on salt. Many foods (even sweet things like fizzy drinks) contain preservatives and flavour enhancers which are sodium-based, so she must look at labels carefully.

Calcium is particularly important for pre-menopausal women to prevent osteoporosis, so she needs adequate amounts of vegetables and some dairy products (not butter!), and perhaps a daily supplement as well. With the help of my recipes (such as Slimmer's Raspberry Cheesecake on page 146) there was no reason why Jaie couldn't carry on entertaining her pals lavishly.

Wine is good for you in moderation, but two bottles at one session is too much. I advised Jaie to switch to spritzers – white wine with fizzy mineral water.

EXERCISE

Nicki: Like so many women who have lost muscle tone after having children, Jaie is particularly concerned about her bulging tummy, so I insisted that she cycled to and from work to increase her calorific output. For the first six weeks her cardio programme was 30 minutes daily, between levels 5 and 6 (brisk walking with intermittent power walking) plus T'ai Chi. I also suggested that she took in a beginners' spinning class (a stationary cycle exercise class designed to provide an intensive cardio workout) and, if possible, a Fab Abs class to help tame her tum!

During the second six weeks Jaie increased her cardio work to 40–45 minutes a day at levels 7–8, and upped the pace. Power walking for two minutes, alternating with 30 seconds of slow jogging, helped build her stamina, and she continued with her Fab Abs and T'ai Chi. With her busy lifestyle I was doubtful whether Jaie would be able to fit everything in. However, as you will find out in Chapter 8, Jaie was a real star and surprised me with her dedication.

ZOË

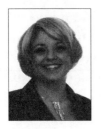

Age: 27	Waist: 29 in
Height: 4ft 11in	Tummy: 30½ in
Starting Weight: 9 st	Buttocks: 38 in
(126 lb/57 kg)	Body Fat %: 18.7%
Job: Beauty Consultant	Blood Pressure: 80/90
Bust: 36 in	Lung Function: 89% (good)

Lovely Zoë lives alone in a flat in Dartford, Kent. She works as a beauty consultant in a large department store in Bexleyheath, Kent. Her mum, Chris, is another of our 'guinea pigs' (see page 31). The family are very close, and Zoë often visits for meals and weekend social gatherings.

Despite the fact that she weighs only 9 st, when we first met Zoë was not happy about her size.

"I am fed up with people telling me that I am not overweight. When you are as short as me, it's horrible being so chubby. I look good at around 8 st, and would dearly love to lose a stone. The only time I achieved it was when I went to the slimming club with mum. We were both doing well, and then my grandfather became ill and neither of us could concentrate on the diet. It all seemed too complicated.

My tummy and bottom look enormous, and although I can hide them behind the counter in the store where I work, I do have to reveal my body, full-length, the rest of the time! I need to slim down to wear anything decent in the evenings.

And I'm not brilliant at preparing meals for one. My fridge tends to be empty apart from a bottle of wine and a couple of ready-meals. I grab a couple of slices of toast and margarine for breakfast, lunch is a jacket potato with tuna, and supper is a plateful of pasta with some cheese on top. Vegetables and salads are a rare treat because it didn't seem worth buying them for one. The only time I get a decent meal is when I visit mum.

Apart from a bit of dancing when I go clubbing with friends, I don't have time to do very much exercise. I tried a step aerobics class, but my co-ordination is so bad that the whole group was stepping one way while I went the other, so I quit. I used to cycle, but I had a knee problem and gave up."

Our Prescription for Zoë

DIET

Sally: Like Lydia, Zoë's lack of energy was due to a very poor diet, which was sadly lacking in iron. It is difficult to get the 'healthy eating' message across to very young people, because it is hard for them to imagine the long-term consequences of inadequate nutrition, but as Zoë wanted to shed some weight as well, this was a great opportunity for her to change her whole approach to the 'chore' of preparing and serving meals.

Her breakfast would be iron-boosted if she chose cereals instead of toast every day, and included some orange juice to aid iron absorption. She needed to make time to buy her own fruit and vegetables, perhaps from a market near her work. Entertaining her mum for a change would give her an incentive to cook more imaginative meals. A wok would be a good investment for cooking quickie meals such as stir-fries. Ready-meals are fine occasionally, but do need a boost with fresh salads and vegetables to add more vitamins and minerals.

Zoë also needed to drink more water. In a job which entails long hours standing in a hot store, fluid needs are increased. If she could stock up that empty fridge with some mineral water and lemons to make a refreshing drink, it would help her diet considerably.

EXERCISE

Nicki: Zoë is so tiny that every inch shows ... especially when it's around the behind! Walking on a gradient (up hills or on a treadmill at the gym) would help tone her backside, and increase her heart rate as well. For the first six weeks she worked out for 30 minutes at day at Level 5–6,

29

and she added 12 slow lengths at the swimming pool to her routine, plus T'ai Chi.

Most youngsters notice a rapid improvement in performance once they start exercising, and Zoe was no exception. She was soon able to push her workout up to Level 7–8, and added two fast lengths to her 12-length swim, plus a water aerobics class, power walking with light jogging sessions, as well as her T'ai Chi exercises.

CHRIS

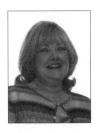

Age: 53
Height: 5ft 1in
Starting Weight: 13 st 2
  (184 lb/84 kg)
Job: Hairdresser
Bust: 42½ in

Waist: 37½ in
Tummy: 43½ in
Buttocks: 42 in
Body Fat %: 24.5%
Lung Function: 77%
(normal)

Unlike our other hairdresser, Lydia, Chris works mainly at home. Her big diet problem is 'picking' from the well-stocked fridge in her kitchen in Dartford, Kent. With her neat blonde bob and immaculate make-up, she looks years younger than her age, but when we met her, Chris felt that her cuddly little body ruined her image.

"When I married my husband Glenn I weighed under 9 st. But 32 years and four kids later, I am bursting out all over. I've been to all kinds of slimming clubs, followed various diets and always ended up fatter than I was before. I seem to have lost confidence in my own ability to stick to any sensible plan. I need nagging all the time.

Two years ago my daughter Zoë and I joined a slimming club and I was thrilled when I lost a couple of stone in six months. But then my dad became ill and I stopped going. Of course, the weight piled back on, with interest.

I dish up big meals for the family, so I am always popping in and out of the kitchen. If there is a half-eaten dish of gateau or a few cold chips in the fridge, it is hard not to gobble them up!

Apart from my daily nibbles, I try to eat fairly sensibly. I have cereal for breakfast, beans on toast for lunch and a big roast dinner or casserole in the evening. I am not a big drinker, but I do enjoy a few glasses of brandy and lemonade when I play darts on Thursday nights.

I feel too self-conscious about my body to go to an exercise class, and my work is at home so I don't even have to walk to and from my job. I can't even use lack of time as an excuse, because my time is largely my own, apart from when the family come round."

Our Prescription for Chris

DIET

Sally: The key to Chris' diet problems was lack of confidence. After years of trying various diets and going to slimming clubs, she had lost faith in her own ability to eat sensibly for longer than a few weeks at a time. Yet this is a woman who has successfully raised four children, run a home for 32 years, and looks years younger than her real age. This is a very common problem with women like Chris ... nurturing is second-nature to them, 'selfishness' is anathema.

I prescribed a three-month 'cure' which would help Chris lose up to a stone or so, and also re-think her priorities. The first was to put herself first for once. That meant exercising regularly, stocking the fridge with healthy snacks like yogurt (calcium, again, to prevent osteoporosis), salads, dried fruits, and telling the whole family that they must support her. If they decided to descend when she was planning to go swimming, tough!

She was also eating far more fatty food than she thought, especially at night and during weekends. Preparing low-fat meals for a change would do the family good, and why couldn't they, occasionally, do their own cooking? Keeping a food diary was an important part of Chris's plan, and she got together with Zoë so they could help each other with their new lifestyle.

EXERCISE

Nicki: Chris loves swimming, so incorporating it into her workout was obviously a good idea. For older women (admittedly, Chris looks far younger than her age!), one advantage is that swimming is easy on the joints, and cools the body down, making exercise appear less tiring than a land workout of similar difficulty.

For the first half of the three-month programme, Chris exercised for 30 minutes daily at moderate intensity (Level 5–6) and took in a water aerobics class, plus slow swimming (12 lengths per session) and T'ai Chi exercises. Power walking on a gradient increased her heart strength. After that she upped the action to 40–45 minutes' exercise at Levels 7–9, and carried on with her T'ai Chi. Power walking was alternated, 50–50, with light jogging.

33

LYNN

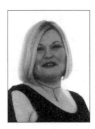

Age: 49	Waist: 45 in
Height: 5ft 6in	Tummy: 49½ in
Starting Weight: 15 st	Buttocks: 46 in
(210 lb/95 kg)	Body Fat %: 36.25%
Job: Beauty Consultant	Blood Pressure: 120/80
Bust: 46 in	Lung Function: 85% (good)

Pretty Lynn was born in Liverpool but moved south to Gravesend, Kent, when her marriage broke up. The split, in 1997, was very traumatic, and made her pile on weight through chronic 'comfort eating'.

When we met up with her, she was very, very worried about her size and lack of energy. However, with her history, it was not surprising that she had problems. The challenge, to us, was to help her to become the dynamic, energetic person that she wanted to be.

34

"To look at me, you would never believe that I was once a consultant in a Liverpool slimming club. At the time, I weighed 12 st, but as I have a large frame I looked fairly trim. But when I moved South with my son, who is now 29, my super figure went to pot! I got a terrific job which I still love, and made lots of friends, but my weight piled on.

I start the day fairly sensibly with a cereal and toast-style breakfast, and even eat a healthy sandwich or jacket potato and salad for lunch. But after another sensible meal in the evening, I pig out, eating omelettes, piles of sandwiches and other comforting snacks before bedtime.

I hate myself for doing it, but I can't seem to help it. I have to leave my uniform dress undone at the back, and cover myself with a jacket because I am so large. It is really depressing.

I thought about going to a fitness centre or exercise class, but gave up the idea as a non-starter because of my size. I have no confidence to go to a gym. Imagine walking into a room full of slim people – the very idea gives me the horrors."

Fight Fat, Fight Fatigue

Our Prescription for Lynn

DIET

Sally: Lynn's total calorie intake was about 4,000, but most of it was concentrated at the end of the day ... when she didn't need the food. This meant that her sleep was impaired and she was laying down energy stores which were not needed for activity ... and were therefore readily converted into fat. She is not alone in making this mistake, which accounts for much of the tiredness that people experience in the workplace (and for their wobbly bots!).

There were big energy-sapping gaps earlier on in Lynn's daily diet. She needed to take a break for fruit in the morning, and a drink and perhaps a carbohydrate booster like some dried fruit and a cereal bar in the afternoon. Both would help increase her energy levels and concentration.

Her evening meal could then be something light and delicious like Mexican Baked Fish (see recipe on page 133), or chicken breast with one of the scrumptious salads on page 122–124.

Lynn's danger time was the evenings, when those comfort-food cravings would strike. Keeping a diary of her feelings helped. If she could pin-point just what triggered a binge, she could divert her attention from food with a chatty phone call to a friend, a long hot bath or, in summer, a walk. With her history it is not surprising that she felt the need to turn to food when she was low, but the time had come for her to re-generate her social life. Although her job was her big love, it was time to widen her horizons. An evening class would be fun and get her away from the kitchen.

EXERCISE

Nicki: Lynn's level of fitness was very low, so it was important that she didn't push herself too hard. It does take some time to get used to exercising regularly, so women like Lynn who have quite a bit of weight to lose and are unused to working out must be gentle with themselves. Remember, an injury or strain received when over-training can put you back weeks or months. For the first six weeks, Lynn exercised at Level 5–6 for 30 minutes a day, and did some gentle cycling (on a stationary bike or road bike), and power walking, using her arms to increase momentum and energy expenditure. She also enjoyed my T'ai Chi exercises. After that good start, she was able to increase exercising to 40–45 minutes daily at Level 7–9 four to five times a week, and incorporated 20-second bursts of high intensity work into her cycling programme. Power walking included some light jogging, and she continued with the T'ai Chi exercises. After I took her along to a gym, she realized that not everyone who works out is stick-thin, and actually enjoyed the experience.

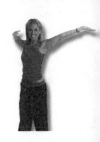

CHAPTER THREE

TIREDNESS AND OVERWEIGHT
– the nutrition connection!

As we've mentioned before, Nicki and I spend many hours answering *Sun* readers' and GMTV viewers' letters and emails, and talking to them on our special Hotline service. Time after time, over-weight men and women tell us that they are deeply unhappy, not solely because of the embarrassment and inconvenience of being fat, but because they lack energy. Ordinary, everyday activities like climbing stairs, running for a bus or lifting up a child for a cuddle are difficult, and sometimes even impossible, because they just don't have the strength to do them.

It's no fun to be fat, and it's definitely no fun to be tired all the time. The two things are inextricably linked together, and in this chapter I am going to tell you why ... and what you can do about it! In Chapter 4 you will try the delicious eating plan which will help you lose weight, and become the energetic, dynamic person you've always wanted to be.

FATIGUE AND SLIMMING

Why did you give up your last slimming attempt? Think about it. Maybe you started on Monday, as most of us do, survived (just!) on Tuesday, felt exceedingly light-headed and tired on Thursday, and reached for a packet of biscuits on Friday. Don't blame your lack of willpower for your failure. There are scientific reasons why you gave up. The tiredness and lack of enthusiasm you felt were very probably caused by a poor intake of nutrients, or a sudden drop in blood sugar – or both.

It's all too easy to miss out on important nutrients when you are trying to shed weight. When you follow a slimming diet, you are taking in less food and fewer calories than you need, and relying on your body to supply the rest. As your body-fat is an inadequate source of vitamins and minerals, it is vital that your weight-reducing diet should be jam-packed with nutrients. Most good slimming-club diets and those published in reputable magazines (and newspapers like *The Sun*) are designed to be healthy, but the sad fact is that some published diets, and the dangerous 'detox' diets that are popular now, are not.

As you will find out when you read the section below, our bodies are like machines which can only work properly when they get the right fuel. If the fuel is poor quality, things start to break down – and one of the first signs that all is not well is tiredness.

Low blood sugar (hypoglycaemia) is also a common problem for slimmers. That sudden energy drop you feel (often just when you need to be energetic; at work, for instance, or when the children are especially demanding), is a physical symptom of low blood sugar caused by long gaps between meals or a sugar or refined carbohydrate 'overload' which causes a 'high' and then a dip in energy and concentration.

Even if they are following a healthy diet plan, many slimmers think they can lose weight more quickly if they cut out meals: skipping breakfast or lunch, for instance. It's not a good idea, because one of the other symptoms of low blood sugar is a sudden desire to eat a sugary or fatty (or both – biscuits are high in sugar *and* fat, so are a top choice for bingers!) food, thus ruining your diet attempt.

If a slimming diet is to work properly – that is, increase your energy for exercise and daily activities, help you to slim and, once you reach your desired weight, stay there – it should follow these criteria:

1 The calorie total should not be too low: 1,500 calories for a woman in a sedentary job, and 1,750 for a man, also in a sitting down job, is about right. If you are taking a lot of exercise, you will need extra carbohydrate. Once the desired weight is reached, your calorie intake should be increased gradually (by adding healthy foods, of course ... this is not the time to pig out on junk after all your good efforts!).

2 It should contain a variety of foods which are both healthy and delicious, and have all the nutrients you need to stay in top form. (See the list below.) It should also include the five portions of fruit and vegetables which the Government recommends for good nutrition and to help prevent diseases like cancer and heart disease.

3 Meals and snacks should be very satisfying, and they should be properly spaced out throughout the day, so that there are never long periods when you do not put any 'fuel' in your body.

4 Dishes should be easy to cook, and the foods should be readily obtainable from your local market or supermarket.

5 The diet should fit in with your life – family and relationship commitments, work schedule, etc.

Tiredness and Overweight – The Nutrition Connection

The diet plan in Chapter 4 follows all the rules above. Can't wait to get started? First, please read the rest of this chapter, because the sections below contain information which is vital for you and all your family.

THE NUTRITION 'GOODIES' AND WHAT THEY DO FOR YOU

As already mentioned, 'yo-yo' slimming (bouts of semi-starvation followed by bingeing) causes fatigue through malnutrition. Adequate calories to sustain your daily activities (about 2,000 for non-slimming women, 2,500 for men in sedentary jobs) are obviously very necessary, but what should those calories be made up from? Less than 35 per cent of your daily calories should come from fat, and at least 50 per cent from carbohydrate. Protein should make up the other 25 per cent. In the Western world adults are unlikely to go short of protein, but most of us are eating too much fat and too little carbohydrate.

How can we change the balance of our diet? We all know that we should cut down on fatty meats, high-fat foods such as cakes, biscuits and full-fat cheese, and replace them with foods such as lean meats, fish (especially oily fish), beans, pulses, potatoes and bread. But, in practice, this is hard to do. Traditionally, the protein (usually meat, often containing 'hidden' fat) is the main item on your plate. When this is accompanied by a pile of fatty chips, you can see that the total fat content of your meal can be very high indeed.

Some diet plans actively encourage slimmers to take in more fat and protein because they advise them to reduce carbohydrate. If you cut out potatoes, bread and pasta, you've got to eat something or starve, so you help yourself to a huge plateful of meat. This current fad for very low carbohydrate diets is dangerous because it causes dehydration, puts extra strain on the kidneys, and can lead to health problems including chronic fatigue. Carbs are vital because they convert

40

to glycogen in the body which, in turn, fuels muscles. They are also helpful for slimmers, because, by filling yourself up with low-fat carbohydrate food (including some sweet foods, surprisingly enough), you are less likely to OD on fat.

So, how can we eat more carbs? One way is to make them the central item on your plate ... a jacket potato topped with baked beans, for instance, or a beany hotpot, or pasta. Another way is to boost your daily carb intake with snacks, especially when you are exercising regularly. When you get started on our diet plan you will find it easy to adjust your eating habits to include more carbs.

As you will find out as you read on, the good news is that the nutrients which will help you feel more lively are often present in foods which are low in calories. This means that it is possible to slim and improve your energy levels at the same time, so long as you eat the right balance of foods.

Vitamins

All vitamins are necessary for good health and to help you maintain high levels of energy, but some have a more important role to play than others. Below is a list of vitamins which you should know about before you start your diet. The Government's RDA (recommended daily allowance) of each vitamin is given. These allowances are often discussed by scientists involved in the continual search for 'optimum nutrition'. Many of them feel that our RDA standards in this country are too low. For instance, the RDA for vitamin C (which cannot be stored by the body) is 60 mg, whereas many nutritionists believe that it should be as high as 500 mg. For that reason, beside the Government RDA I have given, where appropriate and in brackets, a figure that many top nutritionists would prefer!

VITAMIN A (RETINOL)

This is an important anti-oxidant, part of the immune system and is vital for bones, teeth, skin and mucous membranes. Long-term deficiency can cause anaemia and thyroid problems, both of which are associated with tiredness.

RDA   800 mcg
Sources   liver, kidney. (Beta-carotene, which is made up of two vitamin A molecules, is in carrots, swedes and dark leafy greens).

VITAMIN B COMPLEX

This group of vitamins work together. They are vital for energy, and as they are all water-soluble and fairly unstable, it is very easy to go short of one or more of them. Deficiency signs include tiredness, poor memory and skin problems, to name just three. Here's a breakdown of the different vitamins that make up this important group.

B1 (Thiamin)

This converts sugars and fats into energy. Without it, you would have no energy at all, so it is critical! Deficiency signs also include increased appetite (even when you are full – which is an important point for slimmers), muscle weakness and, in extreme cases, beri beri.

RDA   1.4 mg (100 mg)
Sources   whole-grain products such as wholemeal cereals and wholewheat bread, nuts, seeds, beans, dark green vegetables

B_2 (Riboflavin)

Again, this is vital for energy production. It needs thyroxin to convert into an active form, so if your thyroid gland is underactive, you may need extra Vitamin B_2. Depression, dermatitis and cracked lips, as well as acute lethargy, are just some of the 'nasties' you can suffer if you don't get enough.

RDA   1.6 mg (200 mg)
Sources   wholegrain products, liver, milk, nuts, seeds, watercress, leafy vegetables, green beans, broccoli

B₃ (Niacin)

Although the body can make a certain amount of this, you need some spare vitamin B_2 and B_6 (important for pre-menstrual problems), so it's wise to make sure you get enough. If not, your body will just slow down; you could suffer muscle weakness, depression, poor concentration.

RDA   18 mg (450 mg)
Sources   whole grains, liver, meat, poultry, fish, vegetables

B₅ (Pantothenic acid)

This is another vital nutrient for energy. It works with the other members of the B group to maintain good health. A lack of this vitamin (and/or any of the others in the group) will have a detrimental effect on mood, behaviour, mental powers. This vitamin is also vital to fight infection.

RDA   6 mg (500 mg)
Sources   wholegrains, liver, egg yolks, milk, nuts, seeds, vegetables

B₆ (Pyridoxine)

This one helps metabolize protein, break down stored glycogen and keep you feeling perky. It is also involved in the metabolism of iron, which is essential for energy. If you are on the Pill, or suffer pre-menstrual tension, you need extra B_6. One test of whether you are getting enough is good dream recall, as it is involved in the brain's ability to store dream information! Nasties that can arise through lack of this vitamin include carpal tunnel syndrome, dermatitis, eczema and other skin problems.

Tiredness and Overweight – The Nutrition Connection

RDA   2 mg (7 mg)
Sources   wholegrains, livers, nuts, beans, lentils, green vegetables

Vitamin B$_9$ (Folic Acid)

This is prescribed during pregnancy as it is involved in the correct multiplication of genes (a supplement should be taken before you start your pregnancy, as it is actually very important just before conception), but it is also very important for everyone. It works with iron, so a deficiency can lead to anaemia.

RDA   200 mcg
Sources   wheat germ, liver, dark green leafy vegetables

Vitamin B$_{12}$ (Cobalamin)

Like folic acid, this works with iron to prevent anaemia. It's a good idea to take extra B$_{12}$ whenever you are taking folic acid, as the various symptoms of deficiencies of these vitamins can be confused. Signs include apathy, pale skin, tiredness, and even nerve damage, paralysis and muscle weakness.

RDA   1 mcg (6 mcg)
Sources   meat, fish, eggs, cheese, yogurt

Biotin

This works with enzymes involved in the metabolism of fats, protein and carbs, and is very important for generating energy. If you're not getting enough, your hair can fall out, sleep is affected and you may become very depressed and tired.

RDA   150 mcg (200 mcg)
Sources   egg yolks, liver, brewer's yeast

VITAMIN C (ASCORBIC ACID)

This vitamin, which cannot be stored by the body, is essential for the immune system. Without it you are likely to catch all types of infections, which, in turn, will affect your energy levels. Smokers and drinkers need extra vitamin C, and should take supplements if they are not big fruit and vegetable eaters. As well as poor energy levels, coughs and colds, deficiency signs are bleeding gums, painful joints, stress and, in extreme cases, scurvy. Vitamin C aids iron absorption, helping to prevent anaemia.

RDA   60 mg (500 mg)
Sources   fruits, especially citrus fruits, potatoes, red peppers.
           A boiled egg (iron in the yolk) with orange juice (a good
           source of vitamin C) is a good choice for breakfast because
           the two foods work together ... you top up your vitamin C
           and iron stores at one go!

45

VITAMIN D

Most of the vitamin D in our bodies is formed by the action of sunlight on our skin. It encourages the absorption of calcium from the gut (so is important to help prevent osteoporosis), and has an effect on the immune system. Children and old people are most at risk of low vitamin D levels, especially if they rarely venture outside.

RDA   5 mcg (15 mcg)
Sources   sunlight on skin, vitamin D-fortified dairy products

VITAMIN E

Although not directly concerned in the prevention of tiredness, this fat-soluble vitamin is very important for its anti-oxidant properties. It limits the toxic effects of oxygen on healthy tissues, so is often called the 'anti-ageing' vitamin. Deficiency can affect blood, nervous and immune systems.

RDA   10 mg (260 mg)
Sources   vegetable oils, green leafy vegetables, nuts

VITAMIN K

This is another fat-soluble vitamin, which, although it has no effect on mood and little on the immune system, is extremely important to aid blood-clotting after an injury.

RDA   not established
Sources   green leafy vegetables

Minerals

Minerals are as important as vitamins in your diet, especially as far as the prevention of tiredness is concerned. Here's a guide to four top anti-tiredness minerals.

CALCIUM

Every mother knows the importance of calcium for healthy bones in babies and children and, increasingly, we are becoming aware that calcium is vital for older women to prevent osteoporosis (brittle bones). However, calcium (along with sodium and potassium) is also vital for the correct balance of magnesium in the body, which has been found to be of great importance (see below) in the treatment of chronic fatigue.

RDA   800 mg
Sources   dairy foods, canned fish such as sardines, salmon and pilchards (eaten with bones), broccoli, tofu, soy products

MAGNESIUM

This is found in muscles (where it is needed for the smooth contraction and relaxation of the fibres), bones and nerves, and is important to help energy-forming chemical reactions in the body. So, if you don't have enough, you are likely to feel extremely lethargic and weak. Although severe magnesium deficiency is rare, even a mild deficiency can cause problems. If you drink too much alcohol you can lose magnesium in urine, and some drugs (including water tablets, which are popular with many slimmers) cause depletion as well. Pregnant mums need extra.

RDA   5 mg
Sources   cereals, green vegetables, meat (a small amount), some
           mineral waters

Important Note

A number of studies have taken place using magnesium to treat people with chronic fatigue, with some success. However, if you think this is your problem, it is always a good idea to check with your doctor before taking supplements. A blood test will show whether this is, in fact, the problem.

IRON

Although we don't need a great deal of iron (the body contains about 5 g, which would fit on a teaspoon), it is a mineral which is very difficult to obtain from food, and to absorb. Women of childbearing age lose iron every month during menstruation, and there is now increasing concern that up to a third of all women of this age (especially those following slimming diets) are, to some extent, iron-deficient. Tiredness is a common symptom and, in a severe form, deficiency can lead to anaemia as well. Other symptoms are mouth ulcers, hair loss, brittle nails, poor concentration.

RDA   11.4 mg (adult women who are menstruating); 6.7 mg
           (15 mg) (men and non-menstruating women)
Sources   meat, cereals (especially liver and kidney), eggs, nuts, kidney
           beans

Note

Tannin reduces iron absorption by about two thirds, so try NOT to drink
tea with your iron-rich meals.

ZINC

We need nearly as much zinc as we do iron to stay in tip-top health.
This busy mineral works with about 80 different enzymes in the body,
and they all have an effect on our energy. It's also vital for the production of insulin, the hormone that drives blood glucose into cells
for energy production. If you are not getting enough, you will feel
lethargic and mentally confused or, in contrast, you could experience
hyperactivity. It is connected with reproduction and present in the
male testes, which is why oysters (a good source) and seafood have
the reputation of being aphrodisiacs!

RDA   15 mg
Sources   seafood, especially oysters, seeds, nuts, wheat germ, meat

THE 'BADDIES' THAT SAP YOUR STRENGTH AND RUIN YOUR FIGURE

I've talked about the good things that can help you beat tiredness and lose weight as well. Now we're going to pour a bit of cold water on all this positive stuff, with a list of foods, drinks and bad habits which do the opposite. Don't worry, you will not have to completely give up all the delicious 'naughty' things in your diet. However, you will need to cut back on them if you are to succeed. I've included some easy ways to do so.

SALT

'Baddie' number one is sodium, or salt as it is commonly known. We all eat too much of it, often 'hidden' in packaged foods, but also in things like crisps, peanuts, salty meats, frozen foods and even sweet biscuits and cakes. A high intake causes fluid retention and high blood pressure. So avoid the items above, and read labels to ensure that the foods you choose are not high in salt. Never add salt in cooking (use garlic, herbs and lemon juice instead), and don't add it when you are sitting at the table. Sprinkling salt on food you haven't even tasted is a daft habit.

CAFFEINE

Tea and cola drinks are all stimulants which have a variety of unfortunate effects on your body, including affecting blood sugar levels. The caffeine they contain aggravates headaches and causes insomnia, anxiety and mood swings. Try switching to herbal teas, and drinking more water throughout the day. Don't wait until you are thirsty. Keep a bottle of mineral water with you at all times, and sip when needed. Limit those cuppas to two or three, maximum, each day.

ALCOHOL

Booze, as we have already said, depletes the body of nutrients and contributes to many illnesses. Pity your poor body, as it fights to get rid of alcohol from your system. All that hard work! No wonder you feel exhausted after a boozy night out. It's treacherous for slimmers, too. Booze is calorie-loaded (about 200 for an average half-pint of beer, 100 for a double measure of vodka), so too much of it isn't going to help you slim, or leave you many spare calories for decent, healthy food. A night out on the tiles leaves you dehydrated so, next morning, the scales may indicate that you have lost a couple of pounds. Believe me, they lie! Within hours your body tissues will have re-absorbed water, and your weight will be up again.

I'm not being a killjoy. I recommend the occasional glass of red wine (which contains flavonoids that help protect against coronary heart disease and cancer) and beer (especially stout) which contains some vitamin B and minerals like copper and iron.

FAT

Fat is another 'baddie'. Too much of it leads to obesity and heart disease ... it's hard to feel energetic when your poor arteries are all furred up! The 'Mediterranean Diet' myth that encourages slimmers to slurp oil over everything in sight is misleading, too. ALL fat, from animal or vegetable sources, is high in calories. So use oils and fats very sparingly indeed. Use low-calorie, polyunsaturated fat spreads, and allow just a little oil for cooking and stir-fries. If you use canned tomatoes as a base in your stir-fry or casserole, there is no need to add oil.

LIFESTYLE

It's not just the food and drink we take in that can be bad for our health, it's our terrible eating and drinking habits, too. Late night blow-outs are particularly dangerous ... causing indigestion, weight problems, lack of libido and insomnia. Sadly, most people work hard, over long hours, and use a meal to 'unwind'. If you have this problem, try to reorganize your day so you eat a proper lunch instead of a late dinner. Eat earlier where possible. If you are going out to dinner, make sure you eat sensibly throughout the day so you are not tempted to pig out in the evening.

Special Problems that Cause Tiredness

In this book we aim to help people like our volunteers who are over-weight and tired by encouraging them to eat properly and take more exercise. However, there are some health problems which can cause fatigue and which are very serious, calling for more specialized help. If you suffer (or suspect you suffer) from any of these, talk to your doctor.

ANAEMIA

Severe anaemia may not respond to iron or vitamin supplements. A blood test to measure haemoglobin and ferritin levels is needed. Symptoms may include mouth ulcers, a sore tongue, hair loss, as well as acute tiredness.

DIABETES

One of the symptoms of undiagnosed diabetes is tiredness. In this country many people exist with diabetes without realizing it. If you are very tired, always thirsty, and often need to ' spend a penny', you should go to your doctor. A simple urine and blood test is all you need, and these days treatment is very successful.

IRRITABLE BOWEL SYNDROME AND CANDIDA

Tiredness is just one symptom of both of these problems, but of course there are other important signs as well. IBS can cause bloating, severe stomach cramps, diarrhoea, constipation … or a mixture of all these things. If these symptoms are ruining your life, you must get advice, as simply treating the symptoms (with laxatives, for instance) won't help in the long term.

Candida albicans, or 'thrush' as it is commonly called, has a whole list of symptoms including sore throat, itchiness, skin flaking and cracking, cystitis, diarrhoea, headaches, mood swings, confusion, as well as acute exhaustion. Treatments include pessaries, douching and taking anti-fungal remedies such as garlic. Fermented foods or those containing yeast – such as dairy products, yogurt, bread, beer – should be avoided.

SEVERE PRE-MENSTRUAL TENSION

Many women suffer bloating, tension and fatigue just before a period, and this can be treated by reducing salt in the diet, increasing potassium (found in bananas and orange juice) or taking supplements such as Evening Primrose Oil and vitamin B_6. However, where these symptoms are so severe that a woman is laid up for one week in four, more drastic measures are needed. These days doctors are far more sympathetic to this problem, and can help. So don't suffer unnecessarily.

POST-NATAL DEPRESSION

This is another problem which is now taken far more seriously by doctors. In many cases, good nutrition and Vitamin B supplementation can provide the solution, together with counselling, loving care from relatives, and time. The warning signs are: dog-tiredness, inability to cope, unexplained feelings of inadequacy and antipathy towards baby and family. A healthy diet is vital, so mums with this problem must not, under any circumstances, try to starve themselves back into pre-baby shape.

POST-OPERATIVE FATIGUE

Even after having a tooth out or an ingrowing toenail removed, most people feel tired and run down. After a serious operation such as a hysterectomy, heart or cancer surgery, chronic fatigue can continue for months, or even years. Sometimes, the very same drugs prescribed to help recovery, such as antibiotics, steroids or beta-blockers, can also make you feel very tired and run down. At this time the balance of treatment is vitally important, and your doctor or specialist must help you get back on your feet. Needless to say, good nutrition is top of the list, but sadly many hospitals do not give patients the information they need. Don't forget, you can always insist on seeing a State Registered Dietitian (see page 156).

53

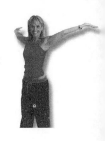

CHAPTER FOUR

YOUR 'SHAPE UP AND WAKE UP' diet plan

This is the great diet plan followed by our six fatigue- and fat-fighting volunteers. It includes everything you need to feel terrific and lose weight. However, before starting any diet plan it is always a good idea to consult your doctor. If you have diabetes or any medical condition which could be affect by a change in diet, then it is absolutely essential that you do so.

The diet is divided into three sections:

1 **The first month's menus eases you gently into a new way of eating, with simple recipes which you can whizz up quickly.**
2 **During the second month you will be increasing the intensity of your daily exercise routine, so there are extra pre- and post-exercise snacks, and the recipes are more inventive to allow you to experiment with dishes which you might not have tried before.**

3   The third month sets the blueprint for good nutrition in the future. It includes plenty of sweet and savoury snacks, and recipes which are elegant enough to be served at a dinner party.

It is safe to follow the diet for as long as it takes you to achieve your 'happy' weight and feel a whole lot more energetic.

DIET PLAN RULES

The plan is suitable for ANYONE who wishes to lose weight. It contains about 1,550 calories daily, is low in fat and has all the vitamins and minerals you need for good nutrition.

If you have over 3 st (42 lb/19 kg) to lose, are taking a lot of exercise or are male, and in a fairly active job, add the Diet Extra foods at the end of each month's meal list.

If you are vegetarian, go for the 'Veggie Option' where indicated.

Daily Allowances

MILK
Your daily milk allowance is half a pint of semi-skimmed, for tea, coffee and to pour on cereals.

DRINK
Half a pint of lager or one glass of dry wine or two pub-measure short drinks daily. Men can have an extra half pint of lager or glass of wine. If you wish you can save up your booze for weekends. Tip: make white wine go further by adding soda water or low-calorie tonic water to make a 'spritzer'. Serve with ice and lemon.

Drink plenty of water – at least six large glasses daily. If you are experiencing severe fatigue it is better not to drink any alcohol at all.

FREE VEGETABLES

You can eat as much as you like of these very low-calorie vegetables, herbs, spices and sauces:

- asparagus
- beansprouts
- broccoli
- Brussels sprouts
- cabbage
- cauliflower
- celery
- lettuce
- mushrooms
- mustard and cress
- pak choi
- peppers (red, green, yellow)
- radishes
- runner beans
- spinach
- spring onions
- tomatoes (canned and fresh)
- watercress
- water chestnuts
- fresh and dried herbs
- garlic
- ginger
- allspice
- curry powder
- Chinese Five spices
- light soy sauce
- Worcestershire sauce
- oriental fish sauce
- lemon or lime juice

Important

Do *not* add salt in cooking or sprinkle it on food.

FIRST MONTH

For the first four weeks you will be easing into the plan. There are no foods on the menus which you cannot buy from your local supermarket. The meals are simple to prepare, and the recipes are a doddle!

Rules

For each day, just choose one Breakfast, one Light Meal, one Main Meal and two Energizing Snacks from the lists below. The snacks can be used as pre- and post-exercise energy-boosters, too. Eat the pre-exercise snack about half an hour before your exercise session, and drink plenty of water. Directly after exercise, choose one of the fruit or cereal bar snacks and, again, nibble with plenty of water. Women with over 3 st to lose and men in fairly active jobs can add the Diet Extras to their daily menus.

tsp	teaspoon
dsp	dessert spoon
tblsp	tablespoon

An asterisk (`) indicates a recipe which can be found in Chapter 8.

Brain-boosting Breakfasts

- 1 packet any cereal from a 'variety pack', milk from daily allowance, small sliced banana, 150-ml glass fruit juice

- 30-g portion porridge oats made up with water, served with a sliced apple, 1 tsp honey and milk from allowance on top

- Slice of wholemeal toast topped with grilled tomatoes, poached egg, watercress, 150-ml glass fruit juice

- Sandwich of two slices wholemeal bread (toasted if you like), 1 dsp (dessert spoon) low-fat cheese spread, sliced tomatoes, lettuce, cucumber, 1 nectarine or pear

- Super Smoothie: blend together small carton natural unsweetened yogurt, 1 small banana, 50 ml concentrated orange juice and a sprinkling of cinnamon. Sip with 1 crispbread spread with 1 tsp jam or marmalade for dunking

- Medium wholemeal roll spread with mild mustard, plus salad and 1 rasher well-grilled back bacon, 150-ml glass fruit juice

- Half a small melon, de-seeded, flesh chopped and mixed with chunks of fresh orange or peach, 2 tblsp any muesli and topped with small carton low-fat fruit yogurt

- Breakfast Fruit Compôte* with 2 tblsp muesli and 1 tblsp low-fat fromage frais or natural yogurt on top

Satisfying Light Meals

- Sandwich of 2 slices wholemeal bread, salad, 50 g lean cold meat or 25 g vegetarian pâté, 1 apple or pear

- Takeaway jacket potato with baked bean or sweetcorn topping, large mixed salad, 1 orange or kiwi fruit

- Large pitta bread stuffed with salad, 50 g prawns or lean cold meat, 2 tblsp cottage cheese, sliced canned asparagus spears or cucumber, lemon juice; small bunch grapes

- Any supermarket sandwich, baguette or flatbread containing 300 calories, plus a 50-calorie fruit drink or 1 apple, orange, pear or peach

- Huge mixed salad from 'free vegetable' list topped with 1 pear, halved and cored with the cavities filled with this delicious mixture: 50 g cottage cheese mixed with 10 g chopped walnuts and a little ground ginger

- 2-egg omelette with filling of canned tomatoes, heated with sliced mushrooms and 1 tsp mixed herbs, huge mixed salad, medium banana

- 200-g potato, baked in microwave or conventional oven with one of these fillings and a huge mixed salad: 25 g camembert cheese mashed with 2 tblsp cottage cheese; 3 tblsp canned red kidney or baked beans; 50 g cooked smoked mackerel mashed with 2 tblsp low-fat cheese spread and plenty of lemon juice and ground black pepper; small can ratatouille and 2 tsp grated parmesan cheese; 1 tsp pesto sauce, cooked spinach

- Heinz 'Big' Soup in any veggie flavour, topped with 1 tsp grated parmesan cheese, served with a small crusty roll, 1 apple or pear to follow

- Pub lunch of chicken or salmon salad or soup of the day with small crusty roll and a small banana to follow

- Cheese and Mushroom Toastie*, 'free' salad, small banana

Family-sized Main Meals

- Turkey with Ginger and Apricot Sauce* or any supermarket turkey or chicken-based ready meal of around 300 calories, 'free' vegetables and salad, sliced kiwi fruit with small carton low-fat fruit yogurt
  Veggie Option: Vegetable Kebabs*, 3 tblsp plain boiled rice, medium (200-g) jacket potato topped with 2 tblsp natural yogurt and lemon juice; apple or orange

- Stir-fry made with 100 g any lean meat (e.g. turkey or chicken breast, pork loin) plus unlimited sliced vegetables, and 2 tsp olive oil; 50 g (dry weight) any noodles with 2 tblsp light soy sauce, lemon juice, garlic and grated ginger to taste; 1 peach or pear
  Veggie Option: use Tofu or Quorn instead of meat

- 110 g salmon steak or other fish fillet, baked in foil with lemon juice, dill or parsley and served with huge portion 'free' vegetables and salad

- Slice of melon with ginger, 50 g any lean, cooked roast meat, thin gravy, 100 g boiled potatoes, huge portion 'free' veggies, Fruit Brulée* or raspberries with 2 tblsp low-fat fromage frais or 1 scoop vanilla icecream
  Veggie Option: serve vegetarian roast cutlet instead of roast meat

- Any 400-calorie supermarket ready-meal with 'free' vegetables and 50 g (dry weight) pasta or rice

- 200 g trout or mackerel, grilled with lemon juice, 200 g boiled or jacket potato, 'free' vegetables and salad, small carton low-fat fruit yogurt
  Veggie Option: serve Quorn instead of fish

- 100 g (dry weight) pasta or rice with sauce made from 500 g jar of Dolmio Light Bolognese Sauce, sliced mushrooms, celery, a few prawns. Serve with a huge mixed salad, and apple or pear for dessert

- Creôle Curry*, 3 tblsp rice, 'free' salad, meringue base topped with sliced kiwi fruit and 1 tblsp low-fat fromage frais or natural yogurt

- 50 g any cold lean meat or 75 g grilled fish, 'free' vegetables and salad, Slimmers' Raspberry Cheesecake*

- 100 g chicken breast, no skin, cooked in the oven in a foil 'parcel' with lemon juice, seasoning, sliced onion, peppers, tomatoes, 'free' vegetables and salad; Apple and Apricot Crumble*

Energizing Snacks

(Choose two)

- 1 small banana

- Meringue nest with raspberries or kiwi fruit

- 6 dried apricots

- Small bunch grapes and 1 crispbread spread with 2 tsp low-fat cheese spread

- Kellogg's Special K or Nutri-grain bar

- 2 jaffa cakes

- Slice of toast spread with Salmon Pâté*

- Bowl of Vegetable and Pasta Soup*

- Small salad roll with mustard or 1 tsp pickle

Diet Extras

(Choose one – for women with over 3 st to lose and men in fairly active jobs only)

- 200-g jacket potato topped with 1 dsp low-fat cheese spread or 2 tblsp baked beans

- Medium salad roll with 50 g lean ham

- Small packet low-fat crisps and low-fat fruit yogurt

- Extra helping from cereal variety pack, topped with large sliced banana and milk from allowance

63

SECOND MONTH

After a month on our diet plan, you are now feeling fitter and livelier. Those awful 'lows' during the day when tiredness seemed to take over your life are becoming less frequent, and you are beginning to enjoy exercise.

The second month of the plan takes into account two facts: first you are burning up more energy and therefore need more carbohydrate and extra water in your plan, and second, you are ready to experiment with more exciting menus and recipes. Don't panic – you won't need to become a telly chef to understand how to cook the delicious dishes I have in store for you! All ingredients are available from your supermarket and there are plenty of choices for vegetarians.

Rules

Follow the list of Allowances given at the beginning of this chapter, and increase water to seven glasses daily.

For each day, choose one Breakfast, one Light Meal, one Supper and three Energizing Snacks from the lists below. Use these as pre- and post-exercise energy boosters and as a nibble when you feel you need extra nutrition and energy – before an evening meeting or during the afternoon, for instance. Women with over 3 st to lose and men in fairly active jobs can add the Diet Extras to their daily menus.

Brilliant Breakfasts

- Savoury French toast: toast one side of a piece of wholemeal bread, spread the other side with 1 tsp low-fat soft cheese, sliced tomatoes, watercress; small glass fruit juice

- Eggy Bread: soak 1 slice wholemeal toast in 1 medium egg, beaten with a little milk from allowance, and fry in a non-stick pan with a light spray of Fry Light; serve with 2 tblsp baked beans, small glass fruit juice

- Fresh fruit salad: slice 1 kiwi fruit, 1 apple and 1 pear served with 1 carton low-fat fruit yogurt on top

- Slice of wholemeal toast topped with small carton (150-g) spaghetti in tomato sauce, sliced tomatoes, watercress; 1 orange

- Banana split: slice 1 small banana horizontally, sprinkle with lemon juice and cinnamon to taste, grill for 2 minutes, then serve topped with 1 carton low-fat fromage frais and 1 tsp chopped nuts

- Sandwich of 2 small slices bread spread with tomato ketchup, watercress, 1 rasher well-grilled bacon or vegetarian breakfast slice; 1 apple to follow

- 30-g portion porridge oats made up with water, served with milk from allowance and 1 carton low-fat fruit yogurt, 1 pear or small banana

65

Luscious Light Meals

- 2 slices wholemeal bread or 1 pitta bread or large wholemeal roll with plenty of 'free' salad and one of these fillings and accompaniments: 2 sardines in brine or oil or 1 tblsp low-fat vegetarian paté, lemon juice, 1 apple; 25 g peeled prawns or low-fat cheese slice or sliced hardboiled egg and 1 tsp low-calorie mayonnaise, a few grapes; 25 g blue cheese, sliced orange, watercress, 1 pear or 2 plums

- 50 g cold cooked chicken, turkey or other lean meat or 75 g grilled fish or canned red kidney or cannelini beans with one of these salads and accompaniments:

- Cheese, Apricot and Walnut Salad*, small wholemeal roll, apple or pear

- Greek Salad*, a few grapes

- Aubergine Salad*, 4 slices canned mango or peach with 1 tblsp low-fat fromage frais

- Large mixed salad from 'free' list, lemon juice dressing, 2 small boiled potatoes, 1 scoop vanilla icecream

- Hot and Spicy Chicken or Tofu Soup*, small wholemeal roll with 1 dsp hummus and salad, 1 satsuma

- Vegetable and Pasta Soup*, small wholemeal roll, 'fun size' choc bar or medium banana

- Avocado Soup*, 2 crispbreads for dunking, 1 orange, a few grapes

- Heinz Big Soup, any flavour, small wholemeal roll, apple, pear or 2 satsumas

- Mug of instant slimmer's soup (about 60–70 calories per sachet), sandwich of 2 slices bread with salad and 50 g cottage cheese with pineapple, small banana

- 250-g jacket potato baked in its jacket in a conventional oven or microwave oven, with large salad from 'free' list and one of the following toppings and accompaniments:

- 50 g cottage cheese mixed with 2 tsp tomato purée or sauce, freshly ground black pepper, small banana

- 100 g smoked haddock, cooked and flaked, 1 dsp low-calorie mayonnaise, cayenne pepper to taste, 1 apple or pear

- 25 g cooked ham, sliced and mixed with 1 tsp Dijon mustard, chopped pear and sliced raw mushrooms, 1 carton diet yogurt

- 2 slices wholemeal toast, with one of the following toppings, side-salad from 'free' list, and accompaniments

- 1 small (150-g) can baked beans, grilled tomatoes, watercress, 1 dsp grated low-fat cheese, a few grapes

- 1 medium egg, poached, fresh cooked spinach or asparagus, lemon juice, black pepper, peach or nectarine

- 1 small (100-g) can tuna in brine or water, mashed and heated with chopped tomato, lemon juice, and garnished with dill or coriander; a few raspberries

- 1 large egg, scrambled with milk from allowance and 25 g smoked salmon (off-cuts are useful for this dish) sliced, garnished with dill, a few grapes

Your Shape Up and Wake up Diet Plan

High-Nutrition Suppers

- Prawn and Almond Salad* or Vegetable and Pasta Soup*, 75 g grilled white fish or vegetarian grill, vegetables from 'free' list

- Large slice melon, Mexican Baked Fish*, 75 g mashed potato, large mixed salad from 'free' list, low-fat fruit yogurt with 3 chopped dried apricots

- 175-g chicken portion, skinned and grilled or roasted, or Caribbean Chicken* or 300 calorie Quorn ready-meal, huge portion 'free' vegetables, Fruit Fool*

- Pasta Primavera*, huge mixed salad from 'free' list, fresh fruit salad made from sliced kiwi, sliced apple, a few grapes and raisins

- Tofu in Tomato Sauce*, 50 g (cooked weight) noodles or rice, huge mixed salad from 'free' list, low-fat fruit yogurt

- Well-grilled beefburger or vegeburger, 75 g oven chips or 200-g jacket-baked potato, grilled tomatoes, watercress, mushrooms poached in chicken or vegetable stock, 3 tblsp peas, huge mixed salad from 'free' list, low-fat fruit yogurt

- Eating Out: any of the following:

- Carvery: melon, lean meat or grilled fish, 'free' vegetables, 1 scoop vanilla icecream, small roll

- Indian: Chicken tikka or tandoori or vegetable curry, salad, 3 tblsp plain boiled rice, 1 poppadum

- Chinese: Crab and sweetcorn soup, Beef in Oyster Sauce, 2 tblsp plain boiled rice, lychees

- Pizza parlour: ½ thin pizza, no extra cheese, large portion of free salad

Energizing Snacks

(Choose three)

- Slice of toast topped with 1 tsp runny honey

- 1 orange

- 2 jaffa cakes

- 2 crispbreads with 2 tsp low-fat soft cheese, watercress, tomatoes

- Small banana

- 4 dried apricots

- Small handful of dried raisins

- Meringue nest topped with frozen raspberries or fresh strawberries and 1 tblsp natural yogurt

Diet Extras

(Choose one – for women with over 3 st to lose and men in fairly active jobs only)

- 75-g portion oven chips and small wholemeal roll

- Large mixed salad topped with 25 g grated hard cheese and 2 tblsp baked beans

- Small packet low-fat crisps and 1 orange and small banana

- 1 bowl cereal from Kellogg's Variety Pack, topped with sliced apple, small handful raisins and milk from allowance

Your Shape Up and Wake up Diet Plan

THIRD MONTH

By now you will have lost up to a stone in weight and feel much livelier. You are becoming used to the idea of eating regularly to 'fuel' your body and brain. Snacking before and after exercise is now part of your routine, and cooking delicious, nutritious meals is fun, not a chore. This month the menus are more flexible: you will enjoy a wide variety of foods and three energizing snacks daily. Even non-veggies will now be enjoying the meat-free dishes.

Remember that the greatest 'convenience' foods are not necessarily things that come in packets. It's quicker and more economical to make a fresh meal from scratch than to fight your way through lots of packaging before heating up a dreary-looking ready-meal. A microwave oven is useful – not just for reheating takeaways but to whiz up delicious breakfasts and puds. I have included some easy recipes (see page 73) which are elegant and delicious enough to be served at dinner parties.

Rules

Follow the list of Allowances at the beginning of this chapter. Sip water constantly throughout the day, not just when you are thirsty.

For each day, choose one Breakfast, one Light Meal, one Main Meal and three Energizing Snacks.

If you wish you can eat the Main Meal at midday and the Light Meal in the evening.

Sustaining Breakfasts

- 2 poached eggs on 1 slice toast, grilled tomatoes and mushrooms poached in a little water, watercress, small glass fruit juice

- Banana sandwich: 2 small slices wholemeal bread, small banana mashed with 1 tsp honey, 1 dsp low-fat natural yogurt, small glass fruit juice

- Stuffed Mega-Mushroom* on 1 slice toast, grilled tomatoes, 1 apple or orange

- Peach and Pear Salad*, 25 g any breakfast cereal, 1 slice toast with 1 tsp jam or marmalade

- 1 packet any cereal from a Kellogg's Variety Pack, milk from daily allowance, 1 carton low-fat fruit yogurt, small glass fruit juice

- 2 rashers well-grilled lean bacon, grilled tomatoes, 2 tblsp baked beans, 1 slice toast, a few grapes

- 30 g portion porridge oats made up with water, milk from allowance, 1 tsp honey or golden syrup, sliced kiwi fruit or a few raisins, 1 carton low-fat fruit yogurt

- Slice toast topped with grilled mango and pineapple slices (fresh or canned) and 1 carton mango or vanilla-flavoured low-fat yogurt

- One-pan hash: pour contents of a 400-g can chopped tomatoes into a non-stick frying pan, add sliced red or green peppers, a few leftover peas, and 25 g any diced cooked meat. Simmer gently for a few minutes, then crack an egg on top of the tomatoes and baste gently until the egg is lightly cooked. Serve straight from the pan with small chunky roll for dunking.

Your Shape Up and Wake up Diet Plan

Healthy Light Meals

- Spanish Omelette*

- 2 slices toast, topped with 1 small can (150 g) baked beans or curried beans or 3 sardines in tomato sauce, salad from 'free' list, 1 apple, orange or pear, 3 dried apricots

- 200-g potato, baked in microwave or conventional oven, with 3 tblsp baked or curried beans with 1 dsp mango chutney and a huge mixed salad

- 1 tortilla, wrapped around the contents of a small, drained can of kidney beans, heated, with drained, canned tomatoes, chilli powder to taste, and topped with 2 tblsp fromage frais and 25 g grated fat-reduced hard cheese. Serve with large 'free' salad, 1 apple to follow

- 200 g salmon or cod fillet, placed on a square of foil and topped with carrots, courgettes and spring onions, cut into matchsticks, plus 2 tsp teriyaki marinade, and lime or lemon juice, freshly-ground black pepper, then baked in a moderate oven (220°C/425°F, Gas Mark 7) for 10–12 minutes. Serve with 'free' vegetables and a small, crusty roll

- Cheese Dip with Fruit*

- Flask of Vegetable and Pasta Soup*, small crusty roll, grilled or roast chicken drumstick (no skin), salad from 'free' list, 1 apple or orange

- Sandwich of 2 slices bread or 2 small slices French bread or pitta bread, with lots of salad and one of these fillings and accompaniments:

- 25 g cold cooked lean meat, 1 dsp sweet pickle, 1 carton low-fat fruit yogurt

- 40 g low-fat cheese spread, 1 orange

- 40 g prawns or other shellfish or 100 g tuna, canned in brine, or 75 g sardines, canned in tomato sauce, with lemon juice and 3 dried apricots to follow

- High Street Eateries and Sandwich Bars:
  Individual Sushi selection pack for one (from supermarkets or Boots Shapers), 1 apple or orange
  Any sandwich, flatbread, pitta or baguette-type packaged snack containing about 350 calories, 1 peach, pear or small banana
  Beefburger in a bun (no onions), huge mixed salad, 1 apple
  Jacket potato with baked bean or coleslaw topping, huge mixed salad, 1 small banana or apple and pear

Sensational Main Meals

- Melon with ginger, Oriental Mackerel*, huge salad from 'free' list

- Chicken Marsala*, 2 tblsp plain rice, 'free' vegetables, small baked apple with 1 tsp honey and 1 tsp raisins

- Tomato and onion salad with lemon juice, basil and garlic, Spiced Leg of Lamb*, 2 tblsp plain boiled rice, 'free' salad and vegetables

- 2 herrings, gutted and coated in seasoned oatmeal, then grilled for 7–8 minutes on each side and served with drained canned grapefruit, chopped, mixed with 3 tblsp plain boiled rice, plenty of 'free' vegetables; 2 scoops fruit sorbet, 1 wafer

- 75 g lean lamb chop or pork tenderloin or Quornburger, grilled and served with 'free' vegetables and side-salad of 3 tblsp canned flageolet beans, drained and mixed with chopped red pepper, crushed garlic, oregano or flat-leaved parsley, freshly ground black pepper, balsamic vinegar to taste; low-fat fruit yogurt

- 2 low-fat sausages (beef, pork or veggie), grilled, cut into pieces and mixed in a pan with canned chopped tomatoes, 2 tblsp baked beans, half a stock cube, garlic, parsley. Heat this chunky 'sauce' and pour over 50 g (cooked weight) any pasta shapes. Serve with 1 tblsp low-fat fromage frais and paprika on top, plus a huge mixed salad from 'free' list

- Stir-fry made with 50 g lean meat, cut into strips, or tofu cut into chunks or 100 g tuna or prawns, plus any fresh, seasonal vegetables from 'free' list, sliced, and light soy sauce, ginger and garlic to taste. Serve with 30 g (cooked weight) pasta or rice and 1 scoop vanilla icecream with a wafer to follow

Energizing Snacks

(Choose three)

- Grilled tomatoes on medium slice toast or soda bread sprinkled with 1 tsp grated parmesan cheese
- Serving of Fruit Fool* with 2 wafer biscuits
- 1 carton cereal from Variety pack with milk
- 1 Kellogg's Special K bar
- 1 Medium banana
- 2 rice cakes with 2 tsps jam and 1 apple

Diet Extras

(Men in active jobs, and women with more than 3 st to lose should choose one each day)

75

- 200-g jacket potato
- 2 slices bread or toast with Marmite or a little low-fat spread
- 3 jaffa cakes
- Small packet low-fat crisps and 1 apple

CHAPTER FIVE

EXERCISE ... WHY IT HELPS
fight fat and fatigue

It's 6 a.m. and the alarm clock is screaming. You know you should get up and start your exercise regime, but you hit the snooze button and vow to pull the trainers on and go for a run after work, when you'll have more energy. Of course, 12 hours later, at the end of an exhausting day's work, you barely have the energy to collapse on the sofa, never mind an hour's roadwork or a trip to the gym.

Perhaps what you need is a long rest, a weekend in bed or a holiday relaxing on the beach in order to preserve the little energy you still have.

Research suggests this is not true.

If you've spent the whole day sitting at a desk, then it's probably your mind, and not your body, that's tired. Even though exercise taxes your muscles and expends calories, it may be just what you need to fight your fatigue. Exercise has a relaxing yet energizing effect which plays a powerful role in relieving feelings of fatigue and exhaustion.

Science has proved exercise to be such a powerful energizer that some doctors have started using it to combat illnesses such as depression and chronic fatigue.

Experts cite a host of physiological and neurological mechanisms that work together to rev up your mind and body. Increased blood flow plays a major part in this revving-up process. When you're at rest – let's say sitting behind a desk or slumped on a couch – your circulation slows down. About three-quarters of your blood remains deep in the core of your body: in your heart, liver, lungs and other internal organs. After a while your body begins to feel sluggish, lethargic and can lower in temperature (especially hands and feet). Essentially, all of your physiological and neurological systems begin to shut down, just as they do when you fall asleep.

However, the moment you step on a treadmill, pick up a skipping rope, strap on skates or dive into a pool, your circulation increases, diverting blood from your core to awaiting muscles in your limbs. As your breathing deepens, life-giving oxygen energizes your muscles and your body becomes invigorated, not only as you work out but for several hours after exercising. Additionally, exercising regularly and achieving a greater level of fitness will eliminate the fatigue that accompanies inactivity. Very fit people have a higher work tolerance. They do not tire as easily when performing everyday tasks such as running for the bus or enduring the flurry of daily challenges. Once you successfully rebuild your energy stores, you will notice increased levels of strength and endurance, and can eventually eliminate fatigue for good.

Expert opinion and the testimony of regular exercisers reveal other benefits that can lessen fatigue. For instance, studies show that people who perform regular, moderate exercise enjoy enhanced immune function and are less susceptible to infection than both sedentary people and ultra-vigorous exercisers – yet, as I will show in the following pages, these are not the only positive effects of exercise.

THE HEALTH BENEFITS OF REGULAR EXERCISE
Mood-affecting Hormones

Exercise triggers emotional and neurological changes which will energize your mind and ward off mood problems that can drain energy. Soon after you begin training, your brain becomes awash with feel-good neuro-chemicals. The elevation of mood during and immediately after exercise may account for the extraordinary commitment and long-term involvement of many exercise fans. Reductions in anxiety and tension, decreases in depression and positive mood changes are no doubt associated with 'feeling better'. Research suggests that changes in the nervous and endocrine systems, brought on by exercise, increase self-confidence.

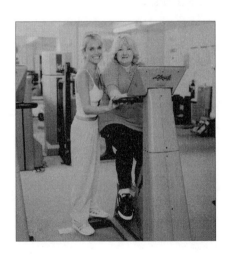

79

Exercise can increase your self-confidence.

The nervous system provides rapid control by fast-travelling nerve impulses, whereas the endocrine system gives slower but more long-lasting control by secretion of hormones directly into the bloodstream, affecting a number of different organs and tissues in a variety of ways. Many hormones are involved in the regulation of energy: epinephrine (also known as adrenalin), cortisol, thyroxine, glucagon and growth hormones all raise blood sugar, resulting in greater energy levels.

Increasing your lung capacity through cardiovascular workouts is vitally important. Insufficient oxygen in the body means insufficient energy, which can result in anything from mild fatigue to life-threatening disease. Unless you have sufficient oxygen in your body, your physical capacity to work effectively will be decreased and your energy and vitality will be drained. However, during exercise or physical activity, adrenalin stimulates the cells into action by supplying oxygen, which generates the production of energy. Additionally, exercise stimulates the release of glucose, thus providing the cells and muscles with a ready energy source. In short, if you exercise regularly, 'feel-good' hormones are released and stress hormone levels plummet, allowing your body to disengage from the energy-sapping fight-or-flight stance it adopts when you are under pressure.

Fat-burning

A sedentary lifestyle is an important factor in the weight-gaining process. It has become increasingly clear that men and women with a physically active lifestyle, or those who become involved in exercise programmes, tend to maintain a good body composition. Evidence is accumulating to support the desirability of an increased level of physical activity. Increased calorific expenditure through aerobic-type exercise is one significant option, resulting in both weight loss and a favourable modification in body composition.

Body composition refers to the relative amounts of fat and lean weight. Although the lean body weight (body weight minus fat weight) is relatively unchanged with exercise, a substantial loss of fat tissue is to be expected.

When exercise is used for fat-burning and weight loss, factors such as frequency, intensity, duration and the specific form of exercise must be considered. Continuous big-muscle, aerobic activities which burn moderate to high numbers of calories – such as walking, running, rope skipping, cycling and swimming – are ideal. Aerobic exercise stimulates lipid (fat) metabolism whereby active, trained muscle is better suited to using fat as a source of energy. The result is improved access to a major source of energy.

Stress and Insomnia

Although the impact of stress on people's lives is still not entirely clear, it appears to be a major factor in mental and physical health, interpersonal relationships and careers. Being 'stressed out' or 'burned out' in one or more areas of life is all too common. Stress is a universal human phenomenon, often causing feelings of distress that have a tremendous impact on behaviour and health. The inability to cope with stress is considered a risk factor for many major health problems such as chronic heart disorders, hypertension, cancer, high blood pressure, ulcers, lower-back pain and insomnia. Although an inability to cope with stress is probably not sufficient, in itself, to cause any of these problems if no predispositions exist, the effects of stress seem to manifest themselves wherever a weak link is found. So, for some people, stress could even result in a cardiac arrest, and for others it could cause insomnia.

Stress can also produce other nasty symptoms. The psychological symptoms can include irritability, poor concentration and short attention span. Behaviour problems include restlessness, severe fatigue, insomnia and loss of sleep. Physiological symptoms can be those associated with the 'fight or flight' reaction, which includes dilation of the pupils, increased heart rate and blood pressure, increased muscle tension, a rush of blood to the muscles and brain and an increased production of catecholamines and corticosteroids, as well as other symptoms not associated with 'fight or flight' such as headaches and back pain.

Happily, the answer to these problems can be found in regular exercise. A recent report by the Centre for Reviews and Dissemination at York University confirmed that 'Specific exercises for back complaints are useful for treating acute low back pain. These include aerobic and muscle relaxing exercises.' Some organizations such as the British Chiropractic Association have long advised *against* bed rest as a treatment for back pain. In most cases, lying flat out can worsen the condition. The muscles begin to atrophy, causing more strain and stress when the sufferer next tries to get up. Light exercise, going about your day-to-day business – and also improving posture by doing yoga, Pilates or T'ai Chi – can help.

As I have already mentioned, exercise combats stress by releasing a cocktail of 'feel-good' hormones into the body whilst lowering stress hormone levels. A well-timed workout (for most people not too close to bedtime) will also aid restful sleep.

PMS (Pre-Menstrual Syndrome)

PMS is a condition that involves a collection of symptoms which regularly occur during the premenstrual phase of a woman's reproductive cycle. Symptoms can include irritability, fatigue, nervousness, depression and other problems which are often distressing enough to affect personal relationships. Increases in follicle-stimulating hormone (FSH), luteinizing hormone (LH) and oestrogen may contribute to the symptoms of PMS. Because the cause of PMS is still unclear, current treatments focus on relieving the symptoms.

Using exercise as a treatment is proving helpful in alleviating the negative moods associated with PMS. Exercise increases blood flow, oxygenation and norepinephrine levels, which can have a beneficial effect on the central nervous system and enhance that 'feel-good' factor.

The Menopause

Menopause is an event that is usually marked by the passage of at least one year without menstruation. The average age at which menstruation ceases is reported to have markedly increased, from about the age of 40 a few decades ago to between the ages of 45 and 50 or even older. The increased susceptibility to osteoporosis among older women is closely associated with the marked decrease in oestrogen secretion that accompanies the menopause. Osteoporosis is the progressive loss of bone mineral mass. The dramatic fall in oestrogen production at the menopause coincides with reduced intestinal calcium absorption, decreased calcitonin (a hormone that reduces mineral loss in your bones) and a decrease in the bones' capacity to re-absorb calcium. The typical woman will lose about 15 per cent of her bone mass in the first decade after the menopause; this increases to 30 per cent by the age of 70. A lack of physical activity hastens this weakening of bones.

Perhaps the most important benefit of regular exercise for women is that it helps to slow down the rate of skeletal ageing. Bones, ligaments and tendons respond to load-bearing exercises. For bones, an increase in activity leads to a denser and stronger structure. The electrical changes created when bone is mechanically stressed stimulates the activity of bone-building, known as osteoblasting. Therefore, exercise of a weight-bearing nature – such as walking, running and skipping – is especially beneficial. Also helpful are activities such as heavy resistance exercises or circuit resistance training, in which significant muscle force is generated against the long bones of the body. So get going, ladies, and build some bone!

FITTING EXERCISE INTO YOUR LIFE

So, you now know all the benefits of exercising regularly, but when can you find the time to do it? Fitting exercise into your busy schedule is not as difficult as it may first appear. It is all about time-management. Let's look at the weekly routine of our 'guinea pig', builder Alan:

Monday to Friday: 6.30 a.m. Rise and get ready for work
7.15 a.m. Travel to work
8.00 a.m –4.30 p.m. Working Day
4.30 p.m. Travel home
5.15 p.m. Make and eat dinner
6.30 p.m. Bathe
7.30–11.30 p.m. Study or watch TV (except on Tuesday evening, when Alan would work out at his local gym)
Saturday: Rise late, pay bills, do shopping, work at gym (p.m.), socialize in evening, late to bed
Sunday: 10 a.m.–7 p.m. Have children for the day. Meet up with friends in evening.

Alan was working out twice a week on average, which was commendable, but he sometimes missed his Tuesday appointment at the gym as he fell asleep after eating his evening meal, and so had slowly been putting on the pounds. I suggested that Alan should exercise at the gym on Mondays, Wednesdays and Fridays, leaving the weekend free for rest and relaxation. In order to resist the temptation of falling asleep when he'd got home and had his dinner, I advised Alan to pack his gym bag on the previous evening, take it to work with him and go for his workout straight from work. I also increased his cardiovascular work in each training session to one hour, with half an hour of weight training. Increasing his cardiovascular training would help to raise his metabolism and burn off fat, and boost his energy levels.

Exercise ... Why It Helps Fight Fat and Fatigue

Alan doubted whether he would have the energy to begin this strenuous regime, so Sally suggested that he eat plenty of carbohydrates on his training days. 'Carb-loading' has long been known to raise energy levels, but it is possible to eat the wrong kind of carbohydrates. White bread, white pasta, white rice and potatoes are difficult for the body to break down, and also have a high sugar content, giving our bodies only short bursts of energy. Steer away from the white carbohydrates and towards the wholemeal alternatives. The most important elements in our diet are fruits, vegetables, pulses and beans, which are rich in the right sort of carbohydrates – that is, they deliver energy over a long period of time without hindering digestion.

With my training advice, Sally's dietary knowledge and Alan's effort, he managed to change his body composition, lose weight and fight fatigue.

You can do it, too!

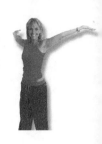

CHAPTER SIX

THE SUPER SIX
– the exercises you need to fight fat and fatigue

O ur six Fight Fat, Fight Fatigue 'guinea-pigs' were each prescribed a fitness routine based around six simple exercises: walking, running, swimming, cycling, skipping and T'ai Chi. *You can follow the same routine.*

Between them, these exercises will help you lose weight, increase your strength and muscle tone, feel less stressed-out and improve your flexibility, balance and co-ordination.

These six key exercises are special because of the vital role they play in effective weight loss and control. Walking (when it's brisk enough), running, swimming, cycling and skipping are all aerobic exercises (which literally means 'with air'). They are more often called cardiovascular exercises these days, as they make your heart work. This is important because, just like any other muscle in your body, your heart needs regular exercise to keep in shape.

I recommend that you choose a combination of these six – say walking, running and swimming, and aim to fit in 30–45 minutes three to five times a week at low to moderate intensity. This is not as difficult as it sounds – for instance, you could go for a really brisk 45-minute walk with your dog on a Saturday afternoon, enjoy a 30-minute swim on Wednesday evening, cycle to work on Friday ('dressed down' in cycling gear, naturally!), and blow away the week's cobwebs with a refreshing, energizing run before Sunday brunch. There ... that's four sessions! Wasn't difficult, was it?

I have also included T'ai Chi because it is a powerful technique which can help boost your self-confidence and inner strength, give you better posture and control and help you relax. That's why I recommend it for everyone. It is particularly useful if you are carrying quite a lot of weight, as the movements are safe and slow and do not require masses of 'puff'.

WALKING

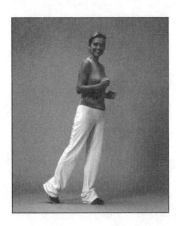

You probably think that you already know how to walk properly ... after all, you do it every day. But let me tell you that, although walking represents our major physical activity, most people don't get enough value out of this enjoyable exercise. Even if you already walk a mile or so a day, there are ways to make your daily walk even more effective.

For a start, you can easily fit more walking into your life. I suggested to all our guinea-pigs that they stopped using their cars for short journeys and walked instead. Or, if they had to use public transport, to walk to the next bus stop along the route.

Next, to turn it into a fat-burning, cardiovascular activity, you need to up the pace. It's been proved that you burn off more calories when you walk faster, so I urged our volunteers to increase their speed levels over a period of weeks until they were 'power walking' – i.e. able to walk fast but still be able to hold a conversation at the same time.

Nicki's Tips for Getting the Most Out of Your Walking

Here are my four top tips for getting the maximum out of your 30- to 45-minute walking exercise:

1 Walk over different surfaces, not just on a smooth pavement. For instance, walking along a sandy beach or through a muddy field (in appropriate footgear!) burns more calories than just walking up the street.
2 Don't be afraid to walk in the snow. It is great exercise and burns off roughly three times as many calories as walking at the same speed on a treadmill.
3 Walk downhill as well as uphill. We all know that an uphill walk increases energy expenditure. Well, the same is true about down-hill walking. This is because extra energy is needed to brake the body (against the downhill pull of gravity) while you maintain a safe walking rhythm.
4 Walking up and down a slope or hill makes the glutes (bottom) muscles work harder, so it can trim your bum as well as help you lose weight.

RUNNING

Jogging and running are becoming more and more popular, as you are probably well aware. If you haven't already taken part in one of the 'fun runs' that take place up and down the country, you could find that starting on my programme will get you hooked!

Running is good news if you have quite a lot of weight to lose, because you will burn off more calories running than walking. The heavier you are, the more calories you burn. However, this has to be balanced out against your ability. It is obviously not a good idea to take up distance running if you weigh 20 st and have never run further than to the end of your road.

Instead, you should aim to get your weight under control (follow our Fight Fat, Fight Fatigue Diet) and start with some easy walking, alternating with longer and longer periods of running as your fitness levels improve.

Once you can run for quite a long way, the benefits are tremendous because you will be effectively burning off fat. At that stage you will notice a distinct change in your body composition ... from flab, to fab!

So, how can running really affect your weight? Well, the average 9½-stone woman will burn 490 calories by running at 5 mph for an hour. As this is enough for a good-sized meal, this is obviously very useful. But is it so boring that you are likely to run straight into the nearest pub?

Some of us can quite happily lace up our trainers, hit the road for an hour-long run and continue this regime for years. However, if the monotony of running makes that intolerable for you, then my 'interval training' (incorporating running and walking at different speeds, plus stretching and resting) will provide you with the interest and variety to keep you stimulated.

New to Running?

Begin your programme with a few 10-minute sessions every day. Simply walk for 100 paces, then run for 100 paces. Three 10-minute sessions will burn as many calories as a 30-minute session and can get you started without putting too much strain on your joints. If you are very unfit, walk all the way – but make it fairly brisk, and try not to stop.

More Experienced?

Once you have mastered the art (and enjoy the pleasure!) of a 30-minute run, it's time to try my hour-long 'interval training' run. This is a winter or summer activity. Just dress appropriately and remember that good footgear is important. No jeans, as they constrict your tummy and thighs and cause cramp.

Don't worry, there are plenty of rest periods, and you can walk if you get tired. Here's the format (remember, you can stop at any time, but you must 'wind down' by walking and, finally, stretching):

Minutes 0–5   Walk, using the posture and technique described in the diagram on page 90.

Minutes 5–10   Stop and stretch your legs, bottom, shoulders and neck.

Minutes 10–12   Walk at an increasingly fast pace, progressing to a steady jog.

Minutes 12–15   Run. In order to burn off 450 calories, you must maintain a steady pace for the duration of the exercise.

Minutes 15–23   Keep running, but now add self-paced intervals of higher-intensity bursts. For example, you could sprint to the third lamppost or tree along your route, then recover with two minutes of jogging. When possible use hills as the most natural form of 'interval'. Between high-intensity periods (which should range in length from 30 seconds to 1–2 minutes), return to a steady running pace.

Minutes 35–40   Slow back down to your jogging pace and add a few short but intense sprints. Really push it as you approach your mental 'finishing line'.

Minutes 40–50   Easy jog, decreasing in speed to a fast-paced walk. Get your breathing back in balance.

Minutes 50–60   Stretch the same muscle groups as you did in the beginning, but hold the stretches for at least 30 seconds.

Nicki's Running Tips

I have eight great tips to help you get the most out of your run:

1 Upright arm posture conserves energy ... so run tall!
2 Keep arm momentum to a minimum during jogging. The arm-pumping action should increase with speed.
3 Legs should swing freely from the hip – the stride that feels the best is usually the most efficient.
4 A heel-to-toe movement is the safest, and less tiring than trying to run on just the balls of your feet.
5 You need proper running shoes with a firm, thick sole, good arch support and a well-padded heel.
6 In winter wear a pull-on cap, as a great deal of body heat is lost through your head.
7 For the first few weeks avoid hard running surfaces. I recommend grassy surfaces or running tracks.
8 To prevent indigestion, discomfort and any tummy cramps, avoid running 1–2 hours after a meal.

93

SWIMMING

Swimming is the ideal exercise for most people because it helps work all the major muscle groups of the body, while the buoyancy of the water prevents damage to the joints. However, you need more than just a gentle splash about in the pool if you are to use swimming as a proper workout.

Ideally, the pool should be just long enough to give a good distance for each length (there's no point swimming just two strokes before you hit your head on the opposite edge of the pool) and spacious enough for you to develop your technique without being jumped on by hordes of screaming schoolchildren.

However, there is no need to be put off if you aren't exactly another Sharron Davis – in fact, a less stylish swimmer burns up more calories over the same distance than an experienced one because they don't cut through the water with the same ease. Even if you are a novice, you can lose weight while treading water – burning off as much as 7.5 cals per minute. Better still, swimming actually burns off more calories per mile than running.

If you are trying to shed weight, don't be put off by worrying about what people at the pool will think of your figure. In my experience, people of all shapes, sizes and ages love to swim. If you do feel a bit lacking in self-confidence, though, it is worth going to the pool early (or late) when you can probably have it to yourself. A bit of research is a good idea before you choose your ideal pool and time for exercise. Aquarobics classes are very popular and effective, so it is always worth checking these out locally. And we mustn't forget – swimming is great fun, too!

Here is my blueprint for the perfect, effective swim:

Poolside		Warm up and stretch.
In the pool	i)	1 length front crawl, 30-second rest.
	ii)	1 length breast stroke, 30-second rest.
	iii)	1 length back stroke, 30-second rest.
	iv)	Tread water for 4 minutes, 30-second rest.

Repeat this routine for as long as you can (don't overdo it), remembering to count the number of strokes you use for each length of the pool. Reducing your stroke count will increase your efficiency. Whether you are a novice or an experienced swimmer, you will benefit from learning how to take fewer strokes per length ... and the good news is that novices improve more quickly than good swimmers.

Nicki's Swimming Tips

Here are my four top tips to help you get in the swim:

1 Whichever stroke you are using, keep your body on an even plane in the water. This will reduce the drag of the water and keep you buoyant.
2 Don't be afraid of being an egghead – wearing a swimming cap makes you go faster and prevents hair damage.
3 Goggles aren't just for show-offs, they protect your eyes and allow you to immerse your head in the water so you get a better gliding action.
4 Beginners can start by swimming widths at the shallow end, gaining confidence before progressing to lengths.

CYCLING

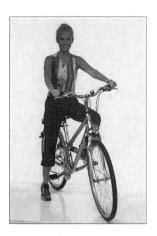

Have you got an exercise bike stashed away in the loft, or a couple of rusting old pedal cycles in the garage? Shame! Cycling is a brilliant fitness and fat-burning exercise. Lots of people who find walking, jogging, running or team sports difficult find that cycling is much easier, and a lot more fun. Of course, the rate at which calories are burned is somewhat slower if you are propelled along on a bike than it is if you are simply using your body as power. In general, you can cycle three to four times the distance covered during a jogging session, and still burn off the same number of calories. However, as you are likely to cover that distance more quickly, it is still an effective and pleasant way to fight the flab.

A typical 9½-stone person will burn about 485 calories cycling at 14–15 mph for 45 minutes. However, the big problem if you are cycling on the road is to motivate yourself to keep going that fast for such a long time, while resisting the urge to coast down every hill. Of course you are also at the mercy of the elements, and sharing the road with cars and heavy lorries can be nerve-wracking.

So, using an indoor bike at home or in the gym or even joining one of the popular 'spinning' cycling classes can be an alternative to cycling on the road. In a recent study, participants in an indoor cycling class burned 7.5–19 calories per minute, totalling 225–570 for a 30-minute session. However, beginners can find these classes too intense and they need to be careful. Don't let an over-enthusiastic instructor intimidate you. A heart rate monitor is useful. Since you are sitting on a stationary bike, reading your heart rate is easy, allowing you to gauge how well you are doing, and thereby improve. Most indoor cycling classes follow an interval programme, with a few minutes spent pushing yourself hard, then periods of recovery, and so on. It's up to you to control the resistance levels on your own bike, and challenge yourself (but not too much!).

How much should you aim for? To improve your cardiovascular fitness you need to cycle continuously for 20 minutes or more, three to four times a week. However, if you are combining cycling with other forms of cardiovascular exercise, this can be cut to once or twice a week. The proper cycling action is a complete circle, pushing down for the first half of the stroke and pulling up with the second, using every muscle in your legs.

Using a Stationary Bike

We've all tried cycling on a stationary bike at the gym or at home at some time or other, so why do so many people give up? It's important to take the 'yawn' factor out of cycling. At home, you can position the bike in front of the telly or in the garden in the summer. In the gym, it's a good idea to take a Walkman with some good music or interesting 'talking book' to keep you entertained.

Depending on your fitness level, try to incorporate 10-second bursts of higher-intensity pedalling, gradually building up to intervals of 30–60 seconds or more. As well as boosting your training level, this will help prevent boredom.

For advanced cyclists: after pedalling away at your normal speed for five minutes, jumpstart your pedalling pace for 20–30 seconds, then drop back down to your regular speed for another five minutes. Repeat these bursts throughout your routine and you will notice a difference in stamina levels after only one month.

97

Getting the Most Out of a Spinning Class

If you are lucky enough to have one of these classes in your area, do have a go. You can pedal your way to a better body – if you follow my advice. Some speed-obsessed spinners might pedal at up to 200 revolutions per minute, yet the professionals reach only 100 to 110 rpm max. If you pedal too fast, one slip of the foot puts huge shearing forces on the knee. What's more, cycling fast doesn't necessarily mean you're burning more calories. For the best calorie burn it's better to crank up resistance and pedal harder, not faster. Stay between 60 and 90 rpm. To calculate speed, count how many circles your foot completes in 15 seconds and multiply by four.

SPINNING DOS AND DON'TS

- DON'T – have the seat too low.
- Adjust the height to fit your leg length. If the seat is too low, your legs remain overly bent, which means you'll pedal bowlegged, slouch and put pressure on the backs of your knees.

- DO – use full leg extension.
- To determine the seat height, sit and push the right pedal down so that your toes and heel are parallel to the floor. Your right leg should be straight with a slight knee bend (10 to 30 degrees). If the seat is too high, your knees will lock and your hips will rock as you pedal, straining your lower back.

- DON'T – do excessive 'jumps'.
- 'Jumps' were introduced when instructors added choreography to basic pedalling. Here, you lift off and on the seat over and over again. This puts extreme stress on your knees, since they bear the brunt of your body weight and you don't burn any more calories.

- DO – stand sporadically.
- It's OK to stand, but don't overdo it. When the instructor yells 'jump!' limit the number of repetitions you do. Keep your back straight, lean your body slightly forward and push your hips back towards your seat. Avoid 'runs', which is standing for prolonged periods while pedalling fast (knee strain is a sign that you've been up for too long). Keep rpm between 60 and 90.

- DON'T – cycle with a super-low body.
- You've seen the super-fit, super-serious rider, crouched down low with a flat back, arched neck and head-to-handlebars stance. Outdoor cyclists do this when racing to glide through wind resistance faster. But there's no wind indoors, so there's no point in putting your lower back in this extremely flexed, stressful position.

- DO – keep your upper body erect.
- Raise the handlebars high enough so that your back is comfortable. Lift your rib cage away from your pelvis to lengthen your spine as you lean forward at a diagonal with a straight back.

- DON'T – flex your hands.
- Rigid hand positions where the wrists remain hyper-extended (palms forward instead of down) can lead to injuries such as carpal tunnel syndrome. A tight grip can put pressure on nerves in the hand and increase blood pressure.

- DO – relax your wrists.
- When seated, you'll find your hands will be most comfortable on the front part of the handlebars, about shoulder width apart. When standing, place your hands on the bar ends, but move them around. Don't force your hands into choreographed positions, it's just not necessary. Do what feels natural and avoid leaning on your wrists.

- DON'T – lock your elbows.
- Some women can't easily rest on the handlebars because many bikes are designed for men, who generally have longer limbs. This and certain hand positions, especially where both hands are touching, can lead to locked elbows, shoulder discomfort and even arm tingling and numbness.
- DO – keep your arms soft.

- If you have to stretch to reach, raise the handlebars, adjust the seat height and move the bike seat forward. Elbows should be soft, not rigid, no matter where you place your hands.

Nicki's Cycling Tips

I have six tips to help you enjoy a 'wheelie' brilliant workout:

1   Adjust the seat height so that your knees are slightly bent at the bottom of a pedalling stroke. No knees under chins, please.
2   Invest in a comfy seat, especially when you are going for a long ride ... ouch!
3   Alternate pedalling strokes – fast and slow – to increase energy expenditure, improve cardiovascular fitness and prevent boredom.
4   When you start cycling, you will find out which muscles are worked hardest during cycling. They are the hip and knee extensor muscles, used during the downward push.
5   Toe clips are useful to help return the pedal to the up position.
6   Always wear a helmet when cycling out of doors.

SKIPPING

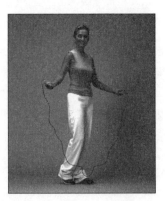

Although I wouldn't recommend skipping as your major exercise, it is a wonderful warm-up or cool-down activity after a run. It is great fun, versatile, and you don't need much equipment. I advise beginners to skip for three sets of three minutes in any one exercise routine. This is because of the stresses skipping can place on the ankles and Achilles tendon. But don't be put off ... even this short workout can tone up your lower body, improve circulation, and burn off those calories.

Fight Fat, Fight Fatigue

Jump Off the Calories

Skipping for three sets of three minutes will burn off nearly 100 calories. Not only that, you can get your heart pumping, feel energized and firm your legs, butt, back and arms. The key is to stay lower but whip the rope faster.

Here's my step-by-step advice on how to get the most out of this high-intensity move:

- To gauge whether the rope is the right length, step in the centre of the rope (part of a washing line will do), handles a couple of inches from your armpits. Stand with your feet about shoulder-width apart, weight on the balls of the feet and heels off the ground. Grip the rope handles lightly, palms facing up.

- Keeping your body upright and knees slightly bent, jump one inch off the ground on the balls of your feet. Swing the rope in an arc, to hit the same spot on the ground as at the start. Practise at a comfortable speed until you can do 30 to 50 repetitions without missing. To up the rope speed, make arm circles as small as possible and flick your wrists on the down stroke. Change your footwork every 30 seconds or so to prevent injury. Some variations: alternate jogging and jumping; twirl the rope around twice in one jump; alternate jumping with your feet shoulder-width, then hip-width apart.

Nicki's Skipping Tips

1 **Rope length: the ends of the rope should reach the armpits when the rope is held beneath the feet.**
2 **Commercial ropes with ball bearings in the handles are easier and smoother to use.**
3 **Skipping requires rapid footwork which will help improve your co-ordination in tennis or other racket ball games.**
4 **Skipping should not be used in the early stages of a fitness programme because of the high impact on ankle, knee and hip joints.**

The Super Six – The Exercises You Need to Fight Fat and Fatigue

T'AI CHI

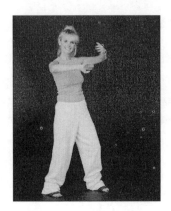

In China, many people start their day with a T'ai Chi session, and this wonderful, relaxing exercise is now becoming very popular in the West. It is the opposite of aerobic activity, because it is slow, controlled and actually decreases the heart rate. So why do I include it in my Super Six? Well, one of the aims of this book is to reduce fatigue levels, and relaxation is an essential part of that process. You can't feel energized if your body is tense and strained, and a daily T'ai Chi routine will help unwind your muscles and soothe your brain. It also helps release tension and reduces health problems such as hypertension, cardiovascular disease and insomnia. So follow my instructions and imagine yourself practising T'ai Chi in the early hours of the morning in Kowloon Park, Hong Kong. Feel that Eastern magic? Of course you do!

General Stance

When standing, your feet should be parallel, shoulder-width apart. Knees should be loose and relaxed. Release the pelvis so that the tailbone points to the ground, which opens up the lumbar region. (This pelvic tilt resembles a pelvis tuck, but don't tense up.) Then lift your spine, and make sure your head is aligned directly over your spine (i.e. not forward, back or to the side). Let your shoulder blades sink towards your hips. Relax your chest, so that you can feel your breath down in your belly.

Movements

Each form consists of various positions that should flow smoothly into each other. The movements should be gentle, without any stress or discomfort.

COMMENCEMENT FORM

1 Stand with your arms down by your side, palms facing back.
2 Raise arms and bend elbows in toward the waist, then circle back out to starting position. Keep hands relaxed.
3 Raise arms, keeping hands relaxed, with palms facing down toward the ground.
4 Lower arms and then stretch arms down, palms parallel to the ground.

BEGINNER'S FORM

5 Turn your hands so that the fingertips point away from the body, as shown.
6 Bring arms in front of your chest with your right hand lower, palm out and your left hand higher and palm facing in. Left foot is forward, with weight on the right foot. Keep your elbows down and start to circle your hands, keeping the movement steady and calm.
7 Turn your body to the right. Step your right foot forward and shift weight to left foot. With right palm up, touch left fingertips to right wrist in 'Hands Play the Lute' position.

103

GRASP THE BIRD'S TAIL FORM

8 Bend knees and turn to the left. Turn right palm in.

9 Shift weight forward and turn body to the right.

10 Continue turning to the right until you make a complete circle, then return to the centre.

11 Shift weight to the right and turn to the left. Change the position of the hands – right palm faces away from the body and left palm faces body, still touching at the pulse.

SINGLE WHIP

12 Open wrists up by bending right wrist over left hand, bringing fingers and thumb together, pointing down. Then turn your left palm towards the body, touching left fingers to right pulse while taking half a step back with the left foot. With the right arm steady and body weight in the right leg, move your left foot back to the centre.

13 Move each arm out to the side, keeping shoulders down. Right hand stays pointed down, while left palm faces out. Each wrist should end up at shoulder height, elbows bent towards the ground with equal weight in each leg. Keep knees slightly bent.

Nicki's T'ai Chi Tips

1 Wear loose-fitting clothes for your T'ai Chi workout.

2 Keep feet bare but make sure you are warm and relaxed.

3 Remember, self-expression is more important than form.

4 Exercise with some relaxing, gentle music.

CHAPTER SEVEN

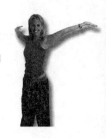

HOW OUR FATIGUE- AND FAT-
fighters shaped up

In Chapter 2 we met the six intrepid volunteers who signed up to try out our Fight Fat, Fight Fatigue programme for three months. They were each prescribed their own routine based on our great diet and fitness plan. They followed it faithfully (some more faithfully than others!), and we caught up with them from time to time to give encouragement.

So, did they lose weight? Do they feel fantastic? Are they now just bursting with energy? Yes, yes and.... wait for it.... YES!

All six members of our FFFF team look and feel a whole lot better than they did when they started the programme. They have achieved a great deal in a short space of time, but it hasn't just been a 'quick fix'. Those are always followed by a downside: a gradual slide back to old, bad habits. Without exception, our volunteers have all made permanent changes to their lifestyles.

Their results prove that the programme really works. All you have to do is follow our advice and you will see results in a very short space of time. What's more, you will enjoy the whole process.

Here's how our gang shaped up:

LYDIA

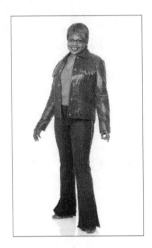

Age: 30
Height: 5ft 2½in
Starting Weight: 11 st 6
 (160lbs/73 kg)
Now: 10 st 7 lb
 (147 lb/67 kg)
Job: Hairdresser

Bust: 39 in
Waist: 33 in
Tummy: 34 in
Buttocks: 38 in
Body Fat %: 36%
Blood Pressure: 130/86
Lung Function: 78%
(normal)

Slimline Lydia loves her gym work.

Hairdresser Lydia was tired all the time when she started our plan, spending every Monday (her day off) in bed recovering from a busy Saturday in the salon and a hectic Sunday spent socializing. Of all our volunteers, Lydia was the most keen on her gym work ... she went, and continued to go, every single day before work.

"I spend 30 minutes on cardiovascular work using the treadmill and rowing machine, and then follow the routine Nicki gave me to strengthen my back. I concentrate on sit-ups with my knees bent, then stretching exercises and T'ai Chi."

Lydia's diet had gone to pot before she started our plan. She kept a food diary for two weeks, and reading through it now is a revelation: she can hardly believe that she ate (and drank!) so badly.

Fight Fat, Fight Fatigue

"On a typical week I would skip breakfast most days, then eat things like a leftover Chinese takeaway for lunch, chicken and chips for supper, and a box of cornflakes washed down with brandy and diet cola as a nightcap. Healthy it was not!"

Now Lydia always eats breakfast before leaving home for the salon; a favourite meal is porridge oats with semi-skimmed milk and banana. Lunch at the salon is a jacket potato with chilli or baked beans and salad, and supper is one of our recipes, such as Spiced Leg of Lamb (page 142) or Spanish Omelette (page 138) with lots of vegetables and salads. She boosts her energy levels by drinking water throughout the day, with nibbles like fruit and rice cakes if she feels droopy.

"I have cut right down on my drinking, too. The occasional glass of red wine is fine, but I now realize how much my drinking habits were interfering with my life: booze definitely saps your energy."

After losing nearly a stone in weight and tightening up her wobbles, she can now wear fashionable skin-tight jeans and trendy tops.

"I love fashionable clothes and was having to squeeze my body into all my outfits … now they are loose. Luckily, the weight and inches seem to have come off my hips and tummy … and my bust is still intact, which my boyfriend is delighted about!"

She is now committed to continuing the programme and aims to shed another stone.

How Our Fighters Shaped Up

ALAN

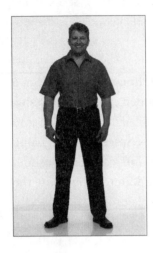

Age: 43
Height: 5ft 10 in
Starting Weight: 14 st 7
   (203lbs/92 kg)
Now: 13 st 8 lb
   (190 lb/86 kg)
Job: Builder and Student

Chest: 42 in
Waist: 34 in
Tummy: 36 in
Buttocks: 37 in
Body Fat %: 20%
Blood Pressure: 140/90
Lung Function: 82% (good)

I feel brilliant!

Alan is a guy who likes to pack a lot into his life, from work and studying to having fun with his three children. When he started the programme he had difficulty fitting everything in, and fitness often came bottom of the list.

"Nicki gave me some motivational strategies, including the simple trick of keeping my gym kit in the car so I never had an excuse to flunk out of my work-out. I used to do just 10–15 minutes of cardiovascular work, now it's 40–50 minutes three times a week, plus weight-training and T'ai Chi – which I love.

   After that lot I feel brilliant and easily up to a bowling session with the children. I just don't feel tired any more."

Alan has definitely achieved his ambition – his 'love handles' have disappeared and he has a 'six pack' chest and well-defined biceps and thigh muscles.

"Nicki told me to work on my lower back as well, to balance the work I've been doing on my stomach. I still want to lose a little bit of fat off my stomach.

Studying takes it out of you, and I'm pleased to report that, after following the FFFF routine, I'm approaching my dissertation on the subject of Charles Dickens with enthusiasm. At this rate I should get my degree some time next year.

I was never a big beer drinker, but food was always my downfall. My favourites were icecream and chips. Now, I cook stir-fries or pasta dishes at home, and have enjoyed the puds on the diet, especially the Fruit Fool (page 148) and Apple and Apricot Crumble (page 147). I eat far more fresh vegetables, have cut out the crisps and eat more fruit. When I eat a bag of crisps now, they taste really fatty. On the whole, though, I eat more than before, just less fat. My taste buds have changed.

My waistline has shrunk by two inches, from a 36 to a 34, and I've had to buy new trousers."

109

Alan's success proves that there is no need for any bloke to succumb to "middle age spread". He looks ten years younger.

JAIE

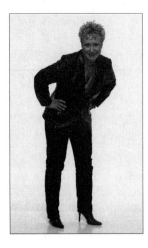

Age: 41	Bust: 36½ in
Height: 5ft 3 in	Waist: 29 in
Starting Weight: 12 st	Tummy: 30 in
(168lbs/76 kg)	Buttocks: 40 in
Now: 11 st	Body Fat %: 35%
(154 lb/70 kg)	Blood Pressure: 84/142
Job: beauty consultant	Lung Function: 80%
	(good)

I'm actually enjoying myself instead of seeing this as punishment … it's a big step for me.

"A couple of weeks after starting our plan, Jaie invested in a trip to Henlow Grange Health Farm which, she thought, would give her fitness campaign a boost. We are sad to report that, despite the luxurious surroundings and fabulous treatments at Henlow, Jaie was not a model guest. In fact, she escaped from the farm and visited the local pub for some wine and a few ciggies!"

After that hiccup, however, Jaie knuckled down and got back on track in establishing a proper relationship with food.

"In the past all my dieting and fitness attempts failed because I'm an 'all or nothing' person who starves herself, then gives up. This time, I've taken it slowly, lost a stone over three months eating delicious meals and taking light exercise, and feel much better.

My brother Malcolm is a superfit member of the local village constabulary, and has been putting me through my paces. Power walking around

Fight Fat, Fight Fatigue

his beat (which includes the local village cemetery) has been fun, and I took Nicki's advice and did my tummy routine every day to beat the bulges. The results are great: I can now get back into my favourite size 14 Dolce and Gabbana jeans, which I haven't worn for years.

I've also taken Sally's advice and cut back on 'hidden' salt in my diet by avoiding things like packaged meals, soups and gravies and, as a result, my fluid retention problems have virtually disappeared. I've cut back on booze, too, drinking 'spritzers' instead of vast quantities of white wine. And I now dish up fresh fruit salad for dessert more often than big, creamy puds.

My favourite recipe on the plan is Créôle Curry (page 143) which is thick and satisfying. I made it recently after we came back from a long walk, and it was yummy: thick and spicy. My reputation as a 'butter mountain' is in tatters since I replaced all butter in my sarnies with a scraping of fat-reduced soft cheese. It tastes delicious and saves loads of calories and fat. Watercress has become my favourite salad vegetable, and I put it in all my sandwiches, too."

Jaie's body fat has gone down from 42.5% to 35% now.

Will Jaie, the original 'yo-yo' dieter, actually stay in shape this time? 'Who knows?' she says, honestly. 'However, I'm actually enjoying myself instead of seeing this as a punishment, which is a big step for me.'

Well done, Jaie ... keep going!

ZOË

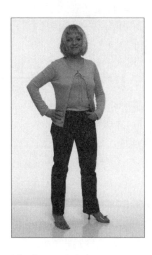

Age: 27
Height: 4ft 11 in
Starting Weight: 9 st
(126lbs/57 kg)
Now: 7 st 12lb
(99 lb/45 kg)
Job: Beauty Consultant

Bust; 34 in
Waist: 25½ in
Tummy: 28 in
Buttocks: 35 in
Body Fat %: 32%
Blood Pressure: 120/90
Lung Function: 92%
(good)

I feel so much more energetic, clothes look better on me and my tum is flat too!

Although she didn't shed the most weight on our programme (her mum, Chris, achieved that honour!), Zoë probably changed her body and lifestyle more dramatically than any of our other volunteers. She now looks absolutely superb, and can wear the size 8 jeans she had hidden at the back of her wardrobe.

"I feel so much more energetic. I look better, too, and clothes, especially tight jeans and cropped tops, look tons better on me. My tum is flat, which is good news, too."

Instead of leaving her fridge empty and relying on fast food and meals with her parents for sustenance, Zoë now plans her week's shopping and cooks up great dishes in her own kitchen using Sally's recipes.

"My fridge is full of fresh salad, vegetables, fruit juice and, of course, the odd ready-meal in case I am in a big hurry. Even if I'm eating alone,

Fight Fat, Fight Fatigue

"I cook pasta, rice, stir-fries – and really enjoy it. My particular favourites are Pasta Primavera (page 136) and Cheese Dip with Fruit (page 124), which is a great Sunday morning breakfast dish – you can eat it and read the papers at the same time.

I've also taken Nicki's advice and increased my daily walking. Before I started, I took the bus into town to work every day. Now I walk there and back, about half an hour each way. My wobbly backside has toned up and I feel energized at work. I am now an account manager at work, and I am sure the FFFF programme gave me the confidence to achieve this promotion."

Dancing has always been one of Zoë's favourite hobbies, and she is now a weekend disco star. 'I always was fond of clubbing, but now they have to drag me off the floor when the place closes,' she laughs.

One of the big bonuses for Zoë is the support of her mum, Chris.

"I would recommend this programme for all ages. Even though we have such different lifestyles, it suits both of us so well. I am so proud of my mum … and I think she's proud of me, too."

113

CHRIS

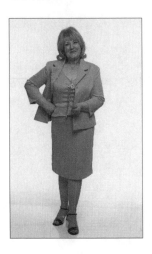

Age: 53

Height: 5ft 1 in

Starting Weight: 13 st 2
(184lbs/84 kg)

Now: 10 st 10
(150 lb/68 kg)

Job: Hairdresser

Bust: 39 in

Waist: 33 in

Tummy: 39 in

Buttocks: 38 in

Body Fat %: 42%

Blood Pressure: 90/148

Lung Function: 82%

Supermum Chris has three other grown-up children besides Zoë, and part of her problem before starting our diet and exercise plan was that she spent a lot of time slaving over a hot stove.

"It was quite difficult to give myself priority, which is something I am sure that a lot of mums my age will understand. But, once I got into the swing of the diet and took time out for exercise, I felt so good that I wanted to carry on. My family have been very supportive and, of course, I have had Zoë's encouragement too. Doesn't she look brilliant?"

Before she started, Chris had resigned herself to being 'chunky':

"I'd lost confidence in myself and decided it was easier to buy skirts with elastic waistbands than lose weight. But this diet and exercise plan is very easy, and rapidly became a way of life."

Chris doesn't drive, so she took Nicki's advice and did plenty of 'power walking' up and down the hills near her home in Dartford, Kent. Chris has three grandchildren, and since losing nearly two and a half stone she has a lot more energy to play with them ... tiredness is no longer a factor in her life.

She has also changed her whole attitude to meal preparation:

"My husband Glenn loves his big meat pies and Sunday roasts. Before I started the programme I would always feel envious when I saw him tucking into a pile of meat on his plate. Now I really don't fancy fatty meals, and heap plenty of vegetables onto my plate instead. I never nibble when I am cooking, either, because I eat so regularly that I'm simply not hungry.

Three months after our diet and exercise plan, Chris went to Manchester to attend her nephew's wedding. 'He is the son of my brother, Alan,' she says. 'Alan hadn't seen me for ages, and was amazed when he saw my new shape.' "

So, did Chris's confidence improve so much that she stayed on our plan? We're happy to report that, more than 12 months after starting her new lifestyle, Chris is still slim and fit.

115

LYNN

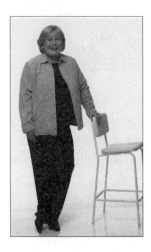

Age: 49	Bust: 43 in
Height: 5ft 6 in	Waist: 40 in
Starting Weight: 15 st	Tummy: 45 in
(210lbs/95 kg)	Buttocks: 43 in
Now: 12 st 12	Body Fat %: 44%
(180 lb/82 kg)	Blood Pressure: 82/121
Job: Beauty Consultant	Lung Function: 89%
	(good)

I've broken the old pattern for good … I feel great!

Lynn's achievement is absolutely tremendous, and she looks great. Even more importantly, she feels brilliant. It wasn't easy for Lynn to break her previous eating habits and improve her fitness level because she was, quite frankly, a very big girl. Once a certain weight is reached, tiredness becomes such a problem that exercise seems out of the question. Lynn could always summon up energy reserves to help her cope with the job she loves as a beauty consultant, but by the end of every working day she was totally shattered, and comfort-ate all evening.

"I've broken the old pattern for good, I'm happy to say. Now, my priorities are different. I actually enjoy the feeling of being fitter and lighter, and I don't want to go back to the old 'me'.

My eating habits are now very different: I have cereal with semi-skimmed milk and fruit for breakfast, and take advantage of the superb restaurant in the store where I work for my lunch and supper. I have a sub-stantial lunch: fish or meat with vegetables, and fruit, then a teatime meal before I go home: beans on toast or a jacket potato, with salad and juice. Instead of pigging out all evening, I drink plenty of water.

Because I've stopped eating so late at night, I sleep soundly and wake early. I go for a walk or do my exercises in the early morning before starting work at 10 a.m. My routine sets me up for the day. I arrive with masses of oxygen in my lungs, and feel great."

Amazingly, Lynn succeeded in losing over 2 st in three months, despite breaking her arm right at the beginning of her Fight Fat and Fatigue campaign:

"I was actually on my way to buy an exercise bike from a friend. She had it in the back of her car, and I stepped into the road to have a look, failed to notice the 7-inch kerb, and stumbled, hitting my arm on the car. Despite this set-back I was able to carry on exercising, and worked out on a tread-mill and cycle in my local gym.

Last summer I went off on holiday to Turkey, and invested in three swimsuits and six sarongs, and a stout pair of walking shoes. I decided that, instead of just lying on the beach, I would spend each alternate day walking in the countryside. I actually managed to shed a few pounds while I was away."

Lynn proves that it is always worth tackling your weight problems, however daunting the task may seem. Just losing 5 kilos and taking more exercise can really improve the quality (and length) of your life.

CHAPTER EIGHT

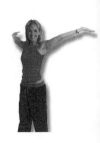

RECIPES

These are Sally's delicious recipes which you need for your Fight Fat, Fight Fatigue diet plan. They are all great for the whole family, as well as slimmers. Enjoy!

The recipes are very easy to prepare. All the ingredients can be bought at your local supermarket. However, it makes sense to shop for the freshest, most reasonably-priced produce you can find. Try farmers' markets and street markets for vegetables, fruit and free-range eggs, and even have a go at growing your own salads and herbs. Even if you only have a window sill or small terrace, it's easy to grow parsley, rosemary, chives and basil in pots and they make a huge difference to the taste of your food.

Equipment is simple too. Don't worry if you don't have a state-of-the-art kitchen (you know the kind: all stainless steel, creamy woodwork and tasteful granite, but far too posh to actually use), because all you need is a grill, an oven, a hot plate or gas ring and some pots and pans. A good, sharp knife is recommended for chopping vegetables and peeling fruit.

When serving up fresh food (even if you are eating alone) always set the table, for example with attractive mats, napkins and fresh flowers. Make surer there is a large salad at main meals (use the "free" ingredients listed on page 57), and plenty of water to drink.

BREAKFASTS AND LIGHT LUNCHES

BREAKFAST FRUIT COMPÔTE

SERVES 4

Calories per serving 150

300 ml unsweetened orange juice
4 tblsp lemon juice
2 tblsp apricot jam
3 firm pears, peeled, halved and cut into sections
8 fresh or dried apricots, sliced
50 g raisins or sultanas
½ tsp cinnamon

120

Put the orange juice, lemon juice and apricot jam into a pan and stir over a gentle heat until the jam has dissolved. Add the fruit and cinnamon to the syrup and bring to the boil, then simmer gently for 12–15 minutes until the pears are tender. Cool slightly or serve cold.

STUFFED MEGA-MUSHROOM

SERVES 2

Calories per serving 170
2 90-g large cap or flat mushrooms
30 g cooked brown or white rice
½ small red pepper, finely chopped
30 g cooked peas or green beans
60 g fat-reduced hard cheese, grated
freshly ground black pepper

Remove the stalks from the mushrooms and chop finely. Mix the chopped stalks, rice, red pepper, peas or beans and pile on top of the mushrooms in an ovenproof dish. Top with the grated cheese, season with pepper and cook in a microwave oven on high for 1½ minutes.

121

PEACH AND PEAR SALAD

SERVES 2

Calories per serving 250

2 medium peaches or nectarines (firm to hard)
2 medium pears (firm to hard)
juice of ½ orange
2 tsp clear honey
150 ml low-fat natural yogurt

Halve peaches, remove stones, cut each half in half again. Cut pears in quarters lengthways and remove cores. Arrange fruit on a plate, pour over orange juice and cook in a microwave oven on high for 4 minutes. Stir honey into yogurt and serve with the warm fruit.

VEGETABLE AND PASTA SOUP

SERVES 4

Calories per serving 130

450 g mixed vegetables, peeled and diced (e.g. carrots, turnip, onions, courgettes, celery, aubergines)
100 g cabbage, shredded
600 ml vegetable stock
300 ml tomato juice
100 g pasta shapes or short noodles
freshly ground black pepper
1 clove garlic, crushed

Place the vegetables in a saucepan with the stock and tomato juice. Bring to the boil, add the pasta, skim, cover and simmer for about 15 minutes, adding seasoning and garlic during cooking.

123

CHEESE DIP WITH FRUIT

SERVES 4

Calories per serving 200
100 g low-fat soft cheese (e.g. Philadelphia Light)
175 g low-fat fromage frais
2 tsp apricot jam
grated rind of 1 lemon
1 tsp ground ginger
8 strawberries or sliced pear, sliced red and green apple, small bunches grapes and cherries, if available

Mix the low-fat soft cheese with the fromage frais, apricot jam, lemon rind and ginger. Spoon dip into a glass dish, chill for 30 minutes, then arrange on a plate, garnished with rind and surrounded by fruity dippers.

CHEESE AND MUSHROOM TOASTIE

SERVES 4

Calories per serving 214

100 g mushrooms
juice of ½ lemon
salt and pepper
100 g carrots
1 small apple
4 thick slices bread
4 100-g slices cheese

Slice the mushrooms, sprinkle with lemon juice, and season. Grate the carrot and apple, and mix with the mushrooms. Toast the sliced bread, top with the mushroom mixture and cheese. Pop back under the grill until the cheese is bubbly.

125

SALMON PÂTÉ

SERVES 6

Calories per serving 50
200 g canned salmon
150 ml plain unsweetened yogurt
1 tsp chopped fresh or dried tarragon or dill
salt and freshly-ground black pepper
squeeze of lemon juice

Drain salmon, remove bones and skin and flake it with a fork, then mash thoroughly. Add the yogurt, tarragon, seasonings and lemon juice to taste. Chill for two hours before serving.

CHEESE, APRICOT AND WALNUT SALAD

SERVES 4

Calories per serving 190 (with dressing)
8 fresh apricots, skinned, or 4 small ripe peaches
    or nectarines, skinned
4 tblsp curd or cottage cheese
100 g walnuts, chopped
salt and freshly ground black pepper
lettuce leaves
1 dsp chopped fresh tarragon or chives
juice of fresh orange
1 tsp oil
1 tsp vinegar

Halve the apricots or peaches or nectarines, and remove stones with a
sharp knife. Mix cheese with walnuts, season to taste, and spoon into the
hollows of the fruit. Arrange on lettuce leaves and sprinkle with herbs.
Make a vinaigrette with the orange juice, oil and vinegar; season to taste.
Pour over the salad just before serving.

127

GREEK SALAD

SERVES 4

Calories per serving 300

1 cos lettuce
½ cucumber, peeled
4 tomatoes, skinned
8 spring onions, trimmed
50 g anchovy fillets (optional)
1 dsp chopped fresh basil
225 g Feta cheese
lemon juice for dressing

Shred lettuce and arrange on a shallow dish. Cut cucumber into 1-inch lengths, cut tomatoes into wedges and arrange on the lettuce. Chop spring onions. Drain the oil from the anchovies, cut into small pieces. Sprinkle the spring onion, anchovy and basil over the salad. Finally, cut the Feta cheese into small dice and pile on top. Squeeze over lemon juice before serving.

128

AUBERGINE SALAD

Serves 4

Calories per serving 40
8 small or 4 medium aubergines
2 tsp olive oil
2 tsp Thai fish or soy sauce
2 tsp light soy sauce
1 clove garlic, crushed
½ tsp brown sugar
2 spring onions, finely chopped
1 tblsp chopped fresh basil or mint
mixed salad greens (e.g. lamb's lettuce, rocket)

Cut the aubergines diagonally into ½-inch thick slices, brush lightly with the oil and grill until browned and soft. Leave to cool. Combine the fish sauce, soy sauce, garlic, brown sugar, spring onions, basil or mint in a bowl and toss the aubergines in the mixture. Leave in a cool place for half an hour to absorb the flavours, then serve on a bed of salad greens.

129

AVOCADO SOUP

SERVES 4

Calories per serving 160

75 ml chicken or vegetable stock
2 ripe avocados, peeled
2 tblsp chopped fresh coriander

Reheat the stock and pour into a blender. Chop one avocado, add to the stock and blend at top speed for 30 seconds. Allow soup to cool to room temperature. Slice the remaining avocado and use as garnish with coriander sprinkled on top. Serve immediately.

HOT AND SPICY CHICKEN OR TOFU SOUP

SERVES 2

Calories per serving 90

750 ml well-flavoured chicken (or vegetable, if using tofu) stock
1–2 small green chillies, seeded and chopped
2 tblsp finely chopped lemon grass
2 kaffir lime leaves or 1 tsp grated lime zest
2 tsp tom yum paste (from Chinese/Asian shops and supermarkets)
100 g drained canned sliced mushrooms
chicken thigh fillet, finely sliced (or 50 g tofu, in small chunks)
2 tsp Thai fish sauce
1 tblsp lime juice
1 tblsp chopped fresh coriander
2 spring onions, sliced

Combine stock, chillies, lemon grass, lime leaves or zest, tom yum paste and mushrooms in a pan and bring to the boil. Cook, uncovered, for five minutes. Add the chicken or tofu, fish sauce and lime juice and simmer for about three minutes. Serve sprinkled with coriander and spring onions.

131

PRAWN AND ALMOND SALAD

Serves 4

Calories per serving 280

400 g fresh cooked, frozen prawns, or 2 200-g cans prawns
350 g can asparagus tips
small jar stuffed green olives
2 tsp olive oil
4 spring onions, chopped fine
3 tblsp tomato purée
juice of 1 lemon
pinch of sugar
3 tblsp tomato ketchup
2 tsp Worcestershire sauce
dash of Tabasco sauce
salt and black pepper to taste
75 g flaked almonds
6 large Webb's lettuce leaves, shredded

Peel the cooked, de-frosted prawns, or drain the cans of prawns and asparagus tips, reserving the liquid. Slice the olives. Heat the oil in a non-stick pan and fry the spring onions lightly for 1 minute. Add the reserved liquid, tomato purée, lemon juice, sugar and sauces. Season to taste, stir and simmer gently for five minutes. Remove from heat, add prawns, almonds and olive slices (save some for garnish). Mix, and allow to cool completely. Leave in the fridge until you are ready to serve. Divide lettuce into six portions, arrange mixture over them, and garnish with the reserved sliced olives and asparagus tips.

FAMILY SUPPERS

MEXICAN BAKED FISH

SERVES 6

Calories per serving 215

1.25 kg haddock fillets
1 lemon, halved
salt and freshly-ground black pepper
3 large cans chopped tomatoes
juice of 1 orange
2 red peppers, de-seeded and sliced finely into rounds
2 small onions, sliced into rings
18 stuffed olives
2 bay leaves
1 tblsp capers, drained
4 sprigs parsley or coriander
2 green chillies, whole or sliced finely
orange slices
parsley or coriander sprigs

Heat the oven to 180°C/350°F/Gas Mark 4. Wipe the fish and rub all over with the lemon; season to taste. Spoon half the canned tomatoes into an ovenproof dish, and place the fish on top. Add the orange juice, peppers, onions, olives, bay leaves, capers, parsley or coriander sprigs, chillies and pour over the remaining chopped tomato. Cover with foil and bake for one hour. To serve, garnish with orange slices and extra sprigs of parsley.

CARIBBEAN CHICKEN

SERVES 4

Calories per serving 320

4 176-g chicken portions, skinned
1 large red pepper, cored, seeded and chopped
1 tsp curry powder
250 ml chicken stock
salt and freshly ground black pepper to taste
4 fresh or canned pineapple rings
1 banana
1 orange, peeled and sliced
watercress

134

Put the chicken portions into a casserole with the chopped pepper and curry powder. Pour over the stock and add salt and pepper. Cover and cook in a preheated oven at 220°C/425°F/Gas Mark 7, for 50 minutes. Chop the pineapple rings and banana and add to the casserole. Cook for a further 10 minutes or until the chicken is tender. Garnish with orange and watercress.

CHICKEN MARSALA

SERVES 2

Calories per serving 280
1 tblsp olive oil
1 small onion, finely chopped
2 cloves garlic, finely chopped
2 100-g boned and skinned chicken breasts cut into thin strips
1 tblsp flour
3 tblsp marsala or sherry
250 ml chicken stock
1 tsp dried tarragon
100 g baby button mushrooms, halved
1 medium red pepper, de-seeded and cut into thin strips
100 g drained, canned sweetcorn kernels
freshly ground black pepper
parsley for garnish

135

Heat the oil in a non-stick saucepan or wok and stir-fry the onion and garlic for two–three minutes. Add the chicken and stir-fry for one–two minutes. Sprinkle the flour into the pan and gradually blend in the marsala or sherry and chicken stock. Add the tarragon, mushrooms, red pepper and sweetcorn. Bring to the boil, stirring well, then reduce heat, cover and cook over a low heat for 15 minutes, stirring occasionally to prevent sticking. Season with freshly ground black pepper and parsley for garnish. This goes well with plain boiled rice or ribbon noodles.

PASTA PRIMAVERA

Serves 4

Calories per serving 170

460 g any pasta or pasta shapes
salt to taste
225 g fresh or canned asparagus
120 g green beans, trimmed
2 carrots, sliced
60 g mushrooms, sliced
1 large can Italian tomatoes
6 spring onions, trimmed and sliced
150 ml low-fat natural yogurt or crème fraiche
freshly ground black pepper
2 tblsp freshly chopped parsley
2 tblsp freshly chopped tarragon

136

Cook the pasta in plenty of lightly salted boiling water, as directed on the packet. Meanwhile, trim any woody ends from fresh asparagus and cut each spear diagonally into 1-inch pieces. Blanch fresh asparagus, beans and carrots for three minutes, then drain well. (If using canned asparagus, slice and add to the other vegetables after cooking.) Place the vegetables and mushrooms into a large pan and stir in the tomatoes and spring onions. Add the natural yogurt, seasonings and herbs and heat gently. When the pasta is cooked, drain well, add it to the vegetable pan and toss to combine all the delicious ingredients. Serve immediately.

TOFU IN TOMATO SAUCE

SERVES **4**

Calories per serving 110

200 g firm tofu

2 tsp oil

4 spring onions, chopped

3 cloves garlic, crushed

3 ripe tomatoes, chopped

1 tsp fish sauce

1 tblsp lime juice

60 ml water

2 tsp tomato paste

2 tblsp chopped fresh coriander

Drain the tofu well, and pat dry with paper towel. Cut into 1- to 1½-inch pieces, brush with oil, then place on a baking tray and grill, turning once, until lightly browned.

Brush non-stick wok with a little more oil, add the spring onions, garlic and tomatoes and stir for three minutes until soft. Add fish sauce, lime juice, water combined with tomato paste, bring to the boil then simmer uncovered for two minutes. Add tofu and coriander to the wok, stir until heated through.

137

SPANISH OMELETTE

SERVES 2

Calories per serving 250
2 tsp oil
½ onion
½ red pepper
½ green pepper, cut into thin slices
90 g cooked potato, diced
60 g cooked peas
3 eggs
3 tsp skimmed milk

Heat the oil in a non-stick pan, and fry the onion and red and green pepper gently until soft. Add potato and peas. Beat the eggs with the skimmed milk, pour into the pan, and cook gently, lifting the bottom of the omelette, so the egg runs underneath. When nearly cooked, brown the top under a hot grill and serve immediately.

ORIENTAL MACKEREL

SERVES 2

Calories per serving 350

2 450-g mackerels, gutted, heads removed
2 rectangles of foil cut large enough to make a loose
    parcel around each fish
1 small onion, peeled
1-inch piece fresh ginger, peeled
350 g tomatoes, skinned and de-seeded
1–2 fresh red or green chilies, seeded
small bunch coriander
freshly ground black pepper

Using a sharp knife, cut the mackerel carefully through the belly from the head to the tail.

Turn the fish, cut side down, onto a board and rub the heel of your hand firmly along the spine. Turn the fish over and lift out the whole of the spine and attached bones. Repeat with the other fish, then wash under cold running water and dry with kitchen paper. Place each fish on foil rectangle. Make stuffing by chopping all the ingredients finely, then season to taste. Spoon inside the fish, then secure openings with long skewers. Fold foil around fish to make a loose but secure parcel. Bake in a moderate oven (180°C/350°F/Gas Mark 4) for 20 minutes and serve garnished with extra coriander leaves.

SPICED LEG OF LAMB

SERVES 4

Calories per serving 350

3-kg (6-lb) leg of lamb, trimmed of fat
3 lemons
10 garlic cloves, peeled
2 x 3-inch pieces fresh root ginger, peeled
1 tsp freshly ground black pepper
1 tsp saffron threads
2-inch cinnamon stick
10 cloves
seeds of 20 cardamoms
2 tblsp clear honey
450 g low-fat natural yogurt
50 g shelled pistachios (optional)
100 g blanched almonds
2 tsp chilli powder
1 tsp turmeric

This one needs to be made the day before you'll want it, due to the long marinating time.

Make deep slashes in the lamb with a sharp knife and place in an ovenproof casserole with a tight-fitting lid. Cut two lemons in half and rub the cut surfaces over the meat, squeezing the juice into the slashes.

Work the garlic and ginger into a paste in a blender or with a pestle and mortar. Add pepper and rub into the meat. Cover and allow to marinate for eight hours. Put saffron threads into a cup and pour over boiling water to cover. Leave to infuse for 20 minutes. Crush the cinnamon, cloves and cardamom seeds with a pestle and mortar. Blend honey, yogurt, pistachios, almonds, chilli powder and turmeric, sprinkle in the crushed cinnamon, cloves and cardamoms. Strain the saffron liquid and mix together. Pour the mixture over the lamb, cover and marinate for a further eight hours.

Place the covered dish into a preheated hot oven (230°C/450°F/Gas Mark 8), and cook for 10 minutes. Reduce temperature to 180°C/350°F/Gas Mark 4 and cook for two hours, basting the meat every 15 minutes. Remove lid, increase oven temperature to hot and cook for a further 10 minutes. Serve hot or cold.

TURKEY WITH GINGER AND APRICOT SAUCE

SERVES 4

Calories per serving 250
225 g dried apricots
2 tsp ground ginger
4 100 g turkey fillets

Place the apricots in a bowl, just cover with water and add the ginger.
Leave to stand for two hours. Place the turkey fillet on the grid of a grill-
pan and spoon over a little of the apricot liquid. Grill for 10 minutes,
turning once. Meanwhile, simmer the apricots for about 10 minutes,
pour into a blender and liquidize. Serve the fillets with the apricot sauce
poured over.

142

CRÉÔLE CURRY

Serves 4

Calories per serving 270
2 tblsp olive oil
2 medium onions, thinly sliced
1 garlic clove, crushed
1 green chilli, de-seeded and sliced
4 small courgettes, cut into ¼-inch slices
1 large red pepper, de-seeded and sliced
3 tomatoes, peeled and chopped
50 g pineapple chunks, canned in juice
1 tsp ground coriander
½ tsp ground cardamom
½ tsp fenugreek
½ tsp turmeric
¼ tsp hot chilli powder
3 tblsp water
275 ml vegetable stock
2 medium bananas, sliced
2-inch slice creamed coconut

143

Heat the oil in a large saucepan over moderate heat. Add onions, garlic, chilli, courgettes and red pepper. Cook, stirring occasionally, for 10 minutes. Add tomatoes and pineapple and cook, stirring frequently, for 10 minutes. Combine spices with water to make a smooth paste, stir into the mixture, then add stock and bananas. Stir in creamed coconut until it dissolves and liquid thickens. Simmer for three minutes. Transfer to a warm dish. Serve immediately.

VEGETABLE KEBABS

Serves 4

Calories per serving 100

1 medium onion, peeled and quartered
4 tomatoes, skinned and quartered
8 button mushrooms
4 courgettes, thickly sliced
1 medium eating apple, cored and cut into eighths
8 bay leaves
Unsweetened apple juice
salt and freshly ground black pepper

Boil the onion quarters for about five minutes until tender but still firm. Thread the onion, tomatoes, mushrooms, courgettes, apple and bay leaves onto four skewers. Place under a pre-heated grill and cook, turning frequently and basting with seasoned apple juice for about 10 minutes.

144

PUDDINGS

FRUIT BRÛLÉE

SERVES 4

Calories per serving 100

450 g soft fruit purée – plums, raspberries, strawberries, rhubarb, black-
berries, etc.
150 ml low-fat fromage frais
4 tsp brown sugar

Place equal quantities of purée in the bottom of four ramekin dishes.
Pour over fromage frais and chill in the freezer for two hours. Sprinkle a
teaspoon of brown sugar over each dish, place under a preheated hot
grill until the sugar bubbles and turns golden. Chill in the fridge for two
hours before serving.

145

SLIMMERS' RASPBERRY CHEESECAKE

SERVES 4

Calories per portion 190

4 size-1 eggs, separated
50 g sugar
25 g plain flour, sifted
2 tblsp very hot water
1 tblsp lemon juice
1 sachet powdered gelatine
900 ml very low-fat soft cheese
½ tsp finely grated lemon rind
fresh or frozen raspberries or strawberries or kiwi fruit to decorate

Line a 9-inch (23-cm) loose-bottomed/springform tin with non-stick paper. Cream the yolks of two of the eggs with half the sugar until very light. Whip the two egg whites until stiff, and, with the flour, fold into the creamed yolks. Spread the mixture evenly in the cake tin and bake in a preheated oven (180°C/350°F/Gas Mark 4) for 18 minutes, until really firm.

Leave to cool, remove from tin, then reline with fresh paper and drop the cake back into the tin. Combine the water, lemon juice and gelatine in a pan of hot water and stir until dissolved. Put the cheese into a bowl and fold in the lemon rind. Whisk the remaining two egg yolks with half the remaining sugar until very creamy. Still whisking, slowly pour in the cooled gelatine mixture. Combine with the cheese.

Whisk the egg whites until firm, add the remaining sugar and continue whipping until stiff.

Carefully, pour the mixture into the cake tin, spreading it over to make the base for the sponge. Chill overnight.

Carefully remove the sides of the tin, and decorate with fruit.

APPLE AND APRICOT CRUMBLE

SERVES 4

Calories per serving 200

500 g sharp eating apples, peeled, cored and chopped
1 tsp lemon juice
75 g dried apricots, soaked overnight and chopped
1 tsp water
½ tsp ground nutmeg
50 g low-fat spread
100 g wholemeal flour
50 g brown sugar

Mix the apples with the lemon juice, apricots, water and nutmeg. Transfer to an ovenproof dish and press down well. Crumble the low-fat spread into the flour with your fingers, then add the sugar, a little at a time. Spread the mixture over the fruit. Place in a preheated oven (180°C/350°F/Gas Mark 4) for 1 hour. Allow to cool before serving.

147

FRUIT FOOL

SERVES 4

Calories per serving 55

225 g puréed strawberries or raspberries, or
      finely chopped fresh or canned pineapple
      or 2 bananas, mashed
300 ml light Greek yogurt
artificial sweetener to taste (optional)

Beat the fruit into the yogurt and spoon the mixture into individual dishes. Chill before serving.

USEFUL ADDRESSES, CONTACTS AND FURTHER READING

Here is a selection of useful contacts and reading from Nicki and Sally's address books. All details are correct at the time of going to press, but do check by telephone or on the appropriate website before writing.

NUTRITION

British Heart Foundation
14 Fitzhardinge Street
London W1H 6DH
020 7935 0185 (you can talk to a cardiac nurse for advice on this number)
www.bhf.org.uk

Diabetes UK
10 Queen Anne St
London
W1M 0BD
Careline: 020 7636 6112
Advice and information for people with diabetes and their families

Disabled Living Foundation
380–384 Harrow Road
London W9 2HU
Helpline 0870 603 9177 (Monday to Friday, 10 a.m.–4 p.m.)
Advice on fitness and diet for the disabled

National Childbirth Trust
Alexandra House
Oldham Terrace
Acton
London W3 6NH
0870 444 8707
Help with diets and pre-natal and post-natal care for new parents and
    their babies

The Vegetarian Society
Parkdale
Dunham Road
Altrincham
Cheshire WA14 4QG
0161 925 2000
www.vegsoc.org
Diet advice and leaflets available

The Vegan Society
Donald Watson House
7 Battle Road
St Leonards on Sea
East Sussex TN37 7AA
01424 427393
Diet advice and leaflets available

Help with Eating Disorders

Promis Counselling Centre
10 Kendrick Mews
London SW7 3GH
020 7581 8222
Free crisis helpline: 0800 374318
www.promis.co.uk
One-to-one counselling and residential treatment (in Kent) for all
     addictive illnesses including eating disorders

National Centre for Eating Disorders
54 New Road
Esher
Surrey KT10 9NU
01372 469 493
www.eating-disorders.org.uk
Telephone counselling and one-to-ones for compulsive and binge
     eaters, bulimics, yo-yo dieters. Counsellors nationwide.

Slimming Clubs

Slimming World

Clover Nook Industrial Estate
Clover Nook Road
Somercotes
Derbyshire DE55 4RF
01773 521111 (classes)
01773 523860 (postal membership)
www.slimming-world.co.uk

Weight Management and Scottish Slimmers

11 Bond Accord Square
Aberdeen AB1 6DJ
0800 362636
Telephone for your nearest class

Weight Watchers

Millenium House
Ludlow Road
Maidenhead
Berks SL6 2SL
08457 123000 (classes)
018628 418500 (postal membership)
www.weightwatchers.com

Websites

Oric (Obesity Resource and Information Centre)

www.aso.org.uk/oric

This site gives all the latest news and research on obesity, worldwide

Weightlossresources.co.uk

On-line database of calories, fat, etc., and can also give you a personalized diet sheet and help.

thesun.co.uk

PO Box 618

Coulsdon

Surrey

CR5 1RU

Regular features and webchats with Sally Ann Voak and other experts' diets and tips.

153

EXERCISE

Reading

E. T. Howley and B. D. Franks, *Health Fitness Instructor's Handbook* (Leeds: Human Kinetics, U.K., 1997)

W. D. Mcardle and F. I. Katch, *Exercise Physiology: Energy, Nutrition and Human Performance* (4th edn; Baltimore, MD: Williams and Wilkins, 1996)

B. J. Sharkey, *Fitness and Health* (4th edn; Leeds: Human Kinetics, U.K., 1997)

J. D. Willis and L. F. Campbell, *Exercise Psychology* (Leeds: Human Kinetics, U.K., 1992)

Gyms and Fitness Centres

The Reynolds Group
The Old Parsonage
113 High Street
Maidstone
Kent ME8 8AA
01634 233194
www.reynoldsgroup.co.uk

This organization has several gyms, including:
Eclipse Fitness Centre
2nd Floor
Westgate House
Spitral Street
Dartford
Kent DA1 2EH
01322 277200
Four of our 'guinea pigs' shaped up at this gym. They also supply personal trainers, work with doctors to help heart patients, and hold dance classes for all levels.

YMCA
Freephone 0845 60 10 728
The YMCA have 33 branches and 87 fitness studios throughout the UK. Fees are very reasonable, and there are concessions for children, young people, seniors and those on low incomes. Excellent YMCA-qualified instructors.

David Lloyd Leisure
0870 8883015

Fifty branches throughout the UK, with membership from £48 per month. Reduced fees for over-sixties. Clubs vary, but usually have high-quality gym equipment and well-qualified staff.

Holmes Place Health Clubs
020 7795 4100

Twenty-four branches throughout the UK. Membership from £40 per month. A wide range of holistic classes, including Yoga and Pilates, as well as the usual gym and fitness classes. A good standard, although free weights are not supplied.

Cannons Health Clubs
0870 780 8182

Over 40 branches and growing all the time. Fees from £40 to £72 per month. Facilities include swimming pools, crèche, etc., but do check before joining as they vary. Instructors all fully qualified.

155

Livingwell Health Clubs
0800 136 636

Seventy-six gyms throughout the UK and Ireland. Membership from £640 per annum. Most clubs have an air-conditioned gym, pool, sauna, etc., and large clubs have hair and beauty salons. Expensive, but they have very well-trained instructors and a thorough new-member-induction programme.

FITNESS AND HEALTH TESTS

Our six volunteers were put through a rigorous fitness test at fitness clubs chosen in conjunction with the FIA (Fitness Industry Association), the UK's leading health and fitness authority. They all meet specified quality criteria, which means that you can join any of them with confidence.

To find out more, check out this website:

www.bupa.co.uk
For information, addresses and links to all the BUPA-approved clubs in your area, should you be interested. Or you could call BUPA on 0207 656 2000.

All addresses and telephone numbers correct at the time of going to press.

INDEX

159

Sun Slimmer

Fight Fat, Fight Fatigue
Firm Up All Over

Nicki Waterman

Firm up all over and discover the fat busting, energizing power of exercise with GMTV presenter Nicki Waterman. Nicki's enthusiasm and empathy for readers is inspirational, and the book provides a terrific range of different routines and workouts so there really is something specially for everyone.

Nicki Waterman, the nation's best-loved fitness guru, shares her guaranteed methods that will take you from fat to fit and from tired out to totally on top of the world by using exercise and key resistance training to gradually re-invent your body.

Full of encouragement for her readers, Nicki understands 'normal' people's worries about fitness. With *Sun Slimmers: Firm Up All Over*, it really doesn't matter if until now you thought brushing your teeth was 'active' or if you're already a regular gym goer. One thing's for sure it contains everything you need to know to get back on track and acheive a fabulous, toned and healthy body.

With specific chapters for:

- Upper body – arms, back, cleavage
- Lower body – think thighs
- Buttocks

- Abs (that's your tum)
- Waistline

As :

- 'First Steps' ultra easy plan to get you started.
- 'Write Your Own Prescription' based on body type and your favourite activities.
- Special tips for taller and shorter readers.
- Guide to starting a new sport such as running or tennis.

Firm Up All Over is illustrated throughout so all exercises are clear and easy to follow.

The Sun Slimmer

Fight Fat, Fight Fatigue.
Diet & Cookbook

120 EASY RECIPES

Sally Ann Voak

Five tailor-made diet plans from *Sun* columnist Sally Ann Voak so you can follow the one that's right for you, plus 60 fantastic fat-burning, super-energizing recipes. The third book in the Sun Slimmer trilogy

Part 3 of our Sun Slimmer series focusses on food. It contains 5 diet plans complete with energising recipes designed to be delicious, guilt-free and guaranteed to help slimmers see the pounds fall off.

Five versions of the diet are specialised for different sorts of slimmers:

- Lose up to half a stone.
- Lose up to 3 stone.
- Men only diet.
- Teen healthy eating.
- Maintenance diet.

Fatigue and overweight are inextricably linked making the couch-potato comfort-eating option a bit of a lifestyle rut. The Sun Slimmer plan shows how the right foods at the right time of day can make an enormous difference to both your energy levels and your weight!

With weight loss, long lasting energy and health in mind, the recipes have been designed to encourage slimmers to stay on track and include plenty of dishes that you wouldn't normally associate with 'dieting'. Sections include:

- Snacks & Nibbles – healthy boosters to keep the blood sugar steady and keep you going strong. Includes pre- and post-exercise snacks.
- Breakfast – quickie meals that will set you up for the day.
- Packed Lunch – eating on the go.
- Family Suppers – to boost the vitality of every member.
- Dinner Party Dishes – no one will ever guess you're on a diet!
- BBQ's & Picnics – al fresco eating in style.